"This book is set within a period of major change in how people interact with the digital world. Each chapter presents familiar situations and themes that show how social norms are continually questioned and reshaped. Behaviours seen in everyday life, both positive and negative, are clearly mirrored in online spaces. The authors identify key trends and draw on relevant psychological concepts and theories to help explain the challenges facing society and communities, particularly teenagers and those who support them. The book combines analysis with a call to action".

– **Kath Herbert (PhD)**, *Sub-Dean (Learning and Teaching), Charles Sturt University*

"It's a very interesting read. Indeed, I learnt a lot and have adjusted some of my phone settings".

– **Mark Filmer**, *Author of* Three Steel Teeth: Wide Comb Shears and Woolshed Wars

"I think the most important thing to help teens with online safety is education. Telling them to be careful or banning them from doing things online doesn't equip them for the future. I like how the book shows you situations that feel familiar, which made it easier to understand. It made me think differently about what's really going on with people's intentions, how things can easily get out of control and how I respond. It could also help adults to understand how to support us better".

– **A 15-year-old High School Student**

AF865757

Teens and Online Safety

This comprehensive guide equips teenagers and their careers with the knowledge and tools needed to foster safe, responsible, and informed online behaviour. It covers the most pressing cyber safety harms facing young users, such as doxing, cyberstalking, sextortion, catfishing, and online grooming. This book offers practical strategies, real-life scenarios, and evidence-based recommendations to help readers proactively recognise and respond to online threats.

The authors explain how teenagers' digital footprints, privacy settings, and lack of cybersecurity controls can be exploited by malicious actors to launch attacks such as financial theft, social engineering, and doxing. Each chapter includes clear explanations, actionable steps, and expert insights tailored to different audiences. This book also explores the psychological and social impacts of digital interactions to explain how attackers exploit human psychology to manipulate, deceive, or coerce victims into making unsafe decisions. Ultimately, it provides clear, actionable steps for readers to enhance online safety. Readers will develop a holistic understanding of this topic and will be able to apply this to manage their digital footprints, identify and counteract psychological manipulation, and develop strong cybersecurity habits to protect themselves from the harms awaiting them in cyberspace.

This is vital for anyone who works to help teenagers protect themselves online, whether parents or carers seeking to guide them, educators and counsellors looking to integrate digital literacy into their curriculum, law enforcement authorities, or policymakers aiming to develop effective online safety regulations. It is also a valuable tool for students and researchers interested in online safety.

Julie Maclean is a researcher and consultant with over 25 years of experience with strategic technology and psychological research. She holds a Doctorate in Technology. Her research includes the dynamics of online communication and how online behaviours can lead to psychological risks and online threats.

Yeslam Al-Saggaf is a nationally recognised expert in cyber security. He is Professor in Computing at Charles Sturt University, where he has been an academic since 2003. He holds a Bachelor of Engineering (with Honours) in Computer and Information Engineering from International Islamic University Malaysia (IIUM) and a Master of Information Technology and a PhD from Charles Sturt University.

Teens and Online Safety

How to Protect Yourself in Cyberspace

Julie Maclean and Yeslam Al-Saggaf

Routledge
Taylor & Francis Group
LONDON AND NEW YORK

First published 2027
by Routledge
4 Park Square, Milton Park, Abingdon, Oxon OX14 4RN

and by Routledge
605 Third Avenue, New York, NY 10158

Routledge is an imprint of the Taylor & Francis Group, an informa business

© 2027 Julie Maclean and Yeslam Al-Saggaf

The right of Julie Maclean and Yeslam Al-Saggaf to be identified as author of this work has been asserted in accordance with sections 77 and 78 of the Copyright, Designs and Patents Act 1988.

All rights reserved. No part of this book may be reprinted or reproduced or utilised in any form or by any electronic, mechanical, or other means, now known or hereafter invented, including photocopying and recording, or in any information storage or retrieval system, without permission in writing from the publishers.

For Product Safety Concerns and Information please contact our EU representative GPSR@taylorandfrancis.com. Taylor & Francis Verlag GmbH, Kaufingerstraße 24, 80331 München, Germany.

Trademark notice: Product or corporate names may be trademarks or registered trademarks, and are used only for identification and explanation without intent to infringe.

British Library Cataloguing-in-Publication Data
A catalogue record for this book is available from the British Library

ISBN: 9781041158929 (hbk)
ISBN: 9781041158912 (pbk)
ISBN: 9781003681731 (ebk)

DOI: 10.4324/9781003681731

Typeset in Galliard
by codeMantra

Contents

Preface

This book was written to help you stay safer online without asking you to disconnect from the world you live in.

The online world connects you to friends, ideas, and opportunities that previous generations never had. But it also comes with risks that aren't always obvious until something goes wrong.

You've probably been told to "be careful online" more times than you can count. But what does that actually mean? And how do you protect yourself without feeling like you have to give everything up?

This book is here to give you real answers. Because the biggest risks online don't come from technology alone, they come from how people use it. From manipulation and pressure, to moments where something feels "off" but is hard to explain. These situations can happen to anyone, no matter how smart, confident, or experienced they are online.

That's why this book focuses on helping you to:

- Recognise what's really going on beneath the surface
- Understand how people influence and manipulate online
- Make decisions that protect you and the people around you
- Build confidence and resilience

Think of this book as something different. It's designed for teens, using real-world situations, to help you understand online risks and feel more prepared to manage them. You can't avoid being online, but with the right knowledge, you can be safer.

Preface

Acknowledgements

This book was shaped by the voices and experiences of young people.

To the teens who shared their perspectives, challenges, and questions, thank you. Your honesty about what it's really like to grow up online shaped not just what this book says, but how it says it.

You made it clear that you don't need more lectures. You need clarity, honesty, and tools that make sense in your world. Your feedback challenged assumptions, highlighted what matters most, and kept this book grounded in reality.

This book is stronger because of you, and it is for you.

Introduction

Why a book on teens and online safety?

A recent study we conducted, funded by the eSafety Commissioner, found that almost all high school students aged 14–18 own a smartphone and spend substantial time online. Our findings also revealed that many teenagers adopt a careless approach to online safety, and a significant proportion of young participants engage in risky smartphone behaviours.

Additionally, a 2024 eSafety study of 1,799 teenagers found that four in ten had negative experiences while gaming online. The risks teenagers face in the digital space are real. The Australian Centre to Counter Child Exploitation (ACCCE) received 82,764 reports of online child sexual exploitation in 2025. This compares with 58,503 reports in the previous year, representing a 41% increase. These statistics underscore the growing threats teenagers face online.

The ACCCE report also highlighted that females are more vulnerable to harmful cyber-safety incidents than males, with a higher likelihood of experiencing unwanted contact and exposure to inappropriate content. Our recent study further revealed that female participants had a lower understanding of key technology concepts compared to their male counterparts.

While the Australian Government has introduced legislation to protect teenagers online, and the eSafety Commissioner provides effective reporting mechanisms, awareness remains a challenge. According to the ACCCE, more than 50% of parents and carers are unaware of these resources, making it unlikely that teenagers are fully informed about them.

In response, the Australian Government has launched initiatives such as the *Act Now. Stay Secure* campaign, which aims to educate the broader community about simple, everyday actions people can take to stay safe online and build cyber resilience, including using strong passphrases and multi-factor authentication, keeping devices updated, and discussing online safety openly with family and peers. Even when teenagers and parents are well-informed, there is a general reluctance to report incidents of cyber-harm or seek help, underscoring the need for awareness efforts that are both accessible and destigmatising.

DOI: 10.4324/9781003681731-1

Ensuring teenagers feel safe online requires proactive support. Raising awareness among both teenagers and parents using language that resonates with them will empower them to navigate cyberspace safely. This book aims to equip teenagers and parents with the knowledge needed to recognise and respond to online threats. Using accessible and relatable language, it explains common cyber dangers such as cyberbullying, trolling, radicalisation, and hate speech.

The book also explains how teenagers' digital footprints, privacy settings, and lack of cybersecurity controls can be exploited by malicious actors to launch attacks such as financial theft, social engineering, doxing, cyberstalking, sextortion, catfishing, and online grooming.

How is this book structured?

This book provides a structured approach to digital risks for teens. Each chapter follows a consistent structure, including real-life scenarios, prevalence and impact data, psychological and technical perspectives, prevention strategies, and response steps. This method ensures that readers not only understand the risks but also have clear, actionable guidance tailored to their needs.

Each chapter follows this clear and consistent structure, tailored to its specific topic, to ensure teenagers receive the key information they need in a practical and easy-to-follow format:

- **Real-life anecdote:** Each chapter begins with a scenario based on real-life cases to illustrate a teenager's negative online experience.
- **Prevalence:** It then examines how common this experience is among teenagers, drawing on our research or other research with statistics.
- **Psychological manipulation:** This chapter then analyses how attackers exploit human psychology to manipulate, deceive, or coerce victims into making unsafe decisions.
- **Technical analysis:** It explains in simple terms how technological vulnerabilities can be leveraged to execute an attack.
- **Preventive measures:** Readers will learn how to protect themselves or support teenagers technologically.
- **Response strategies:** Finally, this chapter outlines steps to take if one becomes a victim of an attack.

Warning

The book's contents may evoke negative emotions, especially if they trigger memories of bad experiences. Please exercise caution. If at any stage you feel distressed, you are encouraged to stop reading. If you feel you need to talk to someone, please contact a relevant healthcare professional or counsellor or a close friend.

The following sites have excellent resources for support:

Australia: Beyond Blue at https://www.beyondblue.org.au
United Kingdom: Childline at https://www.childline.org.uk
United States: Cybersmile at https://www.cybersmile.org/

What does this book offer?

By increasing awareness among teenagers and parents, this book aims to reduce the risk of online harm. A key outcome is the discussion of clear, actionable steps for teenagers, parents, educators, policymakers, and law enforcement authorities to take to enhance their online safety.

This book is designed to educate, empower, and equip teenagers, parents, caregivers, educators, and anyone interested in online safety with the tools needed to navigate the online world safely. It balances technical explanations with psychological insights, practical solutions, and real-world case scenarios to help readers understand online risks and the strategies attackers use to exploit trust and technology.

By fostering digital resilience, awareness, and informed decision-making, this book aims to create a generation of individuals across all levels of society who can confidently and safely engage in the digital world while advocating for better protections and policies. This book is unique in how it:

1. Highlights the risks teens face online, including cyberstalking, online privacy leakage, cyberbullying, sextortion, mental health, and social engineering, using real-life scenarios.
2. Demonstrates how attackers exploit psychological manipulation and technological vulnerabilities to target victims.
3. Provides clear, actionable steps for teenagers, parents, educators, and those interested in enhancing online safety and responding to cyber threats.

Unlike many existing works that target children of all ages, this book is designed to be practical and easy to navigate, allowing readers to focus on topics relevant to teenagers, who are the demographic most vulnerable to online threats. Its practical and reader-friendly approach enables readers to focus on topics important to adolescents, who are particularly susceptible because they are new to unsupervised online engagement, driven by a strong desire for social interaction and boundary exploration, yet still developing risk awareness.

What is the value of this book?

In today's digital world, teenagers and young people navigate an online landscape filled with both opportunities and risks. *Teens and Online Safety: How to Protect Yourself in Cyberspace* is a comprehensive guide designed to equip teenagers and their carers with the knowledge and tools needed to foster safe, responsible, and informed online behaviour. Covering critical topics such as doxing, cyberstalking, sextortion, catfishing, and online grooming, this book provides a structured approach to understanding and addressing the most pressing cyber-safety harms facing young users today.

This book offers practical strategies, real-life scenarios, and evidence-based recommendations to help readers proactively recognise and respond to online threats. Each chapter includes clear explanations, actionable steps, and expert insights tailored to different audiences. Readers will learn how to manage their digital footprints, identify and counter psychological manipulation, and develop strong cybersecurity habits to protect themselves from the harms awaiting them in cyberspace. The book also explores the psychological and social impacts of digital interactions, ensuring a holistic understanding of online safety.

This resource is ideal for adolescents looking to protect themselves online, parents seeking to guide their teens, educators looking to integrate digital literacy into their curriculum, law enforcement authorities wanting to update their understanding of how cyber criminals targeting teens think, and policymakers aiming to develop effective online safety regulations and support. It will also be a valuable tool for students and researchers interested in online safety, online privacy, and cybersecurity.

What topics does this book cover?

The content spans a wide range of topics. This breadth ensures that readers gain a well-rounded understanding of the risks associated with being online and the tools to navigate it safely. While teenagers will find guidance on how to protect themselves, parents and educators will gain tools to support young people, and policymakers or law enforcement authorities will receive insights into how these challenges can be addressed at a broader level.

Introduction

This chapter introduces the book as a practical guide to recognising, preventing, and responding to online harms. It blends real-life scenarios, research-based insights, and actionable steps to equip readers, such as teenagers, parents, educators, and those interested in online safety, with the knowledge they need to navigate digital risks safely. Each chapter introduces a specific online threat and follows a structured approach: a real-life scenario illustrating the issue, research on its prevalence, an analysis of how attackers manipulate trust and emotions, an explanation of the technical aspects involved, prevention strategies, and clear steps on how to respond.

Part 1: Building digital awareness and protection

These chapters introduce fundamental concepts to help develop a strong foundation in online safety.

Chapter 1 – Being aware of your digital footprint

Every action online leaves a trace, shaping digital identities that can impact future opportunities, reputations, and personal security. This chapter explores how posts, shared content, and interactions contribute to a long-term digital presence. It provides teenagers with guidance on managing their digital footprint, while also equipping them with strategies to embrace responsible online behaviour and the importance of digital literacy.

Chapter 2 – Smartphone settings and your identifying information

Smartphones leak vast amounts of personal information, making them a primary target for privacy breaches and cyber threats. This chapter examines how social engineering tactics can be used through smartphone apps to manipulate teens into sharing information that puts their personal safety at risk. It explores how teenagers can manage their smartphone privacy and security settings to control personal information and location data exposure. It covers key security features, such as app permissions, location tracking, and personal information leakage.

Chapter 3 – Protecting your privacy to prevent and mitigate cybersecurity attacks

Online privacy extends beyond smartphones and affects every aspect of digital life. This chapter examines broader cybersecurity risks such as phishing scams, identity theft, cyber-attacks, and the social engineering tactics used to execute them. Additionally, it highlights the dangers of sharing identifying information, whether knowingly or unknowingly, through photos, videos, metadata, and social media activity, offering practical steps to enhance personal security. It provides guidance on strengthening online security through social media settings, robust passphrases, multi-factor authentication, and secure browsing habits.

Part 2: Online harassment and harmful interactions

These chapters address different forms of online abuse and provide strategies to prevent harm, respond effectively, and support victims.

Chapter 4 – Becoming resilient to cyberbullying and trolling

Online harassment can have serious emotional and psychological effects, whether through targeted bullying or disruptive trolling behaviour. This chapter teaches teenagers how to recognise cyberbullying, respond safely, and seek help to create safe digital environments. It also distinguishes trolling from free speech, offering guidance on promoting positive online interactions.

Chapter 5 – Protecting yourself from cyberstalking and doxing

Persistent online harassment, or cyberstalking, can create fear and distress, particularly when personal information is exposed through doxing. This chapter explains how cyberstalkers operate, how teens can protect their online presence, and how to help victims feel safe. It also provides insight into legal protections and reporting mechanisms for addressing these forms of digital harm.

Part 3: Exploitation and deception

These chapters explore how attackers manipulate trust to exploit, deceive, and bypass security measures.

Chapter 6 – Protecting yourself from sextortion and image-based abuse

Sextortion is a growing threat where young people are blackmailed using explicit images they shared with other people they thought they could trust. This chapter explains the psychological manipulation tactics used by perpetrators and how teens can recognise warning signs before victimisation occurs. It also addresses image-based abuse, outlining legal consequences and resources available for victims.

Chapter 7 – Recognising and responding to catfishing and online grooming

Predators and scammers use fake identities to deceive individuals online. This chapter helps teenagers recognise catfishing attempts, verify online identities, and avoid being manipulated into dangerous situations. It also details online grooming tactics and how predators build trust and isolate victims to help equip teens with the knowledge and skills to detect and prevent exploitation.

Chapter 8 – How to recognise and respond to hate speech and radicalised views

Hate speech and extremist content are prevalent online and can influence young minds. This chapter helps teens recognise and escape harmful content while promoting respectful digital interactions. It also explores how extremist groups advance their agenda and use personal grievances to recruit individuals online. It guides on early warning signs, intervention strategies, and how to prevent radicalisation.

Chapter 9 – How to avoid fake news and online misinformation

False and misleading information spreads quickly online, influencing beliefs, behaviours, and even real-world decisions. The use of AI has exacerbated this phenomenon. AI has made deepfakes more believable and difficult to dispute. This chapter educates teenagers on how to critically assess information, recognise misinformation and disinformation, and verify sources. It also provides tools to foster digital literacy and analytical thinking, while offering insights into the broader challenges of regulating online misinformation.

Part 4: Digital well-being and healthy online habits

These chapters explore how digital experiences affect mental health, offering strategies to balance screen time, reduce harm, and foster resilience.

Chapter 10 – The risks of online gaming

Gaming is an integral part of teenagers' online lives, but it also carries risks such as cyberbullying, scams, and exposure to inappropriate content and other negative experiences. This chapter explores how to create safe gaming experiences, helping teens recognise predatory behaviour and avoid addiction. It provides guidance on monitoring gameplay and fostering positive gaming habits for online gaming safety.

Chapter 11 – Screen time, AI, and mental health

Although online interactions can provide social support, excessive digital engagement can lead to loneliness and social disconnectedness. This chapter explores the balance between meaningful digital and offline connections, helping teenagers develop healthier online habits. It also provides strategies to support teenagers struggling with loneliness and the social connectedness impacts of digital isolation.

Chapter 12 – Using social media and online relationships

Social media plays a major role in self-esteem and mental health. Online relationships also come with risks, including coercion and deception. This chapter provides teenagers with guidelines for safe online interactions and the harmful uses of social media, such as online comparison. It also outlines guidance for online conversations to build healthy online relationships, helping them understand consent in online interactions and avoid exploitation in digital spaces. The chapter also provides tools to support healthy online interactions and strategies to mitigate social media's negative effects.

Who is the audience of this book?

This book is intended for a diverse audience to ensure accessibility for younger readers. It is primarily aimed at teenagers, parents, caregivers, educators, law enforcement authorities, policymakers, and anyone who needs a practical guide to online safety for adolescents. Parents and educators will buy it to help young people navigate digital risks, while policymakers and child-safety advocates will use it to inform broader protection strategies. This book is also relevant for researchers, youth organisations, and online safety trainers.

The book is not specifically aimed at undergraduate or postgraduate students but may be valuable as supplementary reading for courses related to cybersecurity, digital literacy, child protection, cyberpsychology, privacy leakage, and cyber threat education. It can be used in teacher training programmes, high school courses, or online safety seminars and workshops.

This is not a research monograph intended primarily for academic libraries, although it is research-based and may appeal to scholars studying online harm prevention, online safety policies, or cyberpsychology. The subject area for online safety and digital well-being is widely researched and increasingly taught in schools, higher education, and professional training programmes.

This research builds on a recent project funded by the eSafety programme, focused on creating innovative, impactful eSafety initiatives, ensuring inclusivity (especially for children), and promoting the safe use of digital technologies. The project collected real-time data from adolescents on smartphone privacy leakage, knowledge of privacy settings, attitudes towards security settings, and privacy concerns. The research, which adhered to Safety by Design principles, developed effective educational interventions for teenagers. The educational interventions improved teens' knowledge about smartphone privacy leakage. Training sessions were delivered to high school students, IT staff, teachers, and parents in line with the objectives of the Online Safety Grants Program.

This book has strong international relevance, as online safety issues affect teenagers and young people worldwide. While the research and scenarios focus on Australia, the threats and solutions apply to many countries, particularly those with high digital engagement. In addition to Australia, the book is likely to appeal to audiences in the United States, the United Kingdom, Europe, Canada, New Zealand, and other English-speaking regions, as well as international institutions with a regulatory remit and child protection agencies.

This book's foundational coverage of online safety concepts and its structured format make it suitable as an introductory textbook for undergraduate courses in fields like education, psychology, and information technology. Given its practical insights and real-life case studies, this book could also function as supplementary reading for both undergraduate and postgraduate students seeking to deepen their understanding of online safety and digital well-being. While not positioned as a high-level research monograph, the book's comprehensive analysis and inclusion of current digital challenges could provide valuable context and case studies for researchers and academics focusing on cyberpsychology, digital education, or cybersecurity threats.

Who are the authors of this book?

Julie Maclean

Dr. Julie Maclean is a researcher and consultant with over 25 years of experience with strategic technology and psychological research. Her career has been focused on advising businesses on enhancing customer engagement, optimising processes, and integrating advanced technologies to optimise user experience. Her primary focus lies in implementing digital customer experiences that facilitate seamless online interactions, alongside addressing cybersecurity risks and elevating data management capabilities.

Over the past decade, Dr. Maclean has conducted extensive research into the dynamics of online communication, delving into areas such as social media, online privacy, freedom of expression, loneliness, social connectedness, well-being, social rewards, and online photo sharing. Her passion for human-computer interaction drives her exploration of how online behaviours can lead to psychological risks and online threats.

Recently, Dr. Maclean has focused on investigating the cybersecurity threats teenagers face, examining both psychological and technological risks. She holds a Doctorate in Technology, underscoring her commitment to understanding and mitigating the complexities of the digital landscape.

Link to research: https://researchoutput.csu.edu.au/en/persons/julie-maclean/publications/

Yeslam Al-Saggaf

Professor Yeslam Al-Saggaf is nationally recognised as an expert in cybersecurity. His recognition is evidenced by his success in 2022 as the lead Chief Investigator in the Australian Government eSafety Commissioner (eSafety) Grants Program ($87,870). In this project, Professor Al-Saggaf and his research team showed school children how to manage their smartphones' privacy settings to see whether this would empower them to prevent their smartphones from sharing sensitive information. The surveys they conducted before and after the hands-on cyber-safety lessons they delivered to the children revealed that the lessons improved their knowledge, risk attitude, and privacy awareness.

In 2023, Professor Al-Saggaf was also successful as a Chief Investigator in a Cybersecurity Cooperative Research Centre (CRC) grant ($1,350,000). Professor Al-Saggaf's status in cybersecurity is also evidenced by a 2017 invitation from the then Minister for Foreign Affairs, The Hon Julie Bishop MP, to attend the launch of Australia's first International Cyber Engagement Strategy in Sydney. Professor Al-Saggaf has authored numerous publications in cybersecurity, attracting hundreds of citations from scholars. In addition to his interest in cybersecurity, Professor Al-Saggaf is also interested in the phone snubbing phenomenon, commonly known as "Phubbing". His book *The Psychology of Phubbing* (2022) has been acquired by more than 216 libraries worldwide to date and currently has an Altmetric score of 103 (Significant Attention). The book is also available in German.

Professor Al-Saggaf is a *Professor in Computing* at Charles Sturt University, where he has been an academic since 2003. He holds a Bachelor of Engineering (with Honours) in Computer and Information Engineering from International Islamic University Malaysia (IIUM) and a Master of Information Technology and a PhD from Charles Sturt University.

Link to research: https://researchoutput.csu.edu.au/en/persons/yalsaggacsueduau/

Bibliography

Al-Saggaf, Y., & Maclean, J. (2024). Smartphone privacy and cyber safety among Australian adolescents: Gender differences. *Information, 15*(10), 604. https://doi.org/10.3390/info15100604

Australian Centre to Counter Child Exploitation. (2020). *Understanding online child sexual exploitation: Awareness, perceptions, attitudes and preventative behaviours.* Australian Centre to Counter Child Exploitation. https://www.accce.gov.au/sites/default/files/2021-02/ACCCE_Research-Report_OCE_acc.pdf

Australian Centre to Counter Child Exploitation. (2020). *Understanding online child sexual exploitation: Awareness, perceptions, attitudes and preventative behaviours: Factsheet.* Australian Centre to Counter Child Exploitation. https://www.accce.gov.au/sites/default/files/2021-02/ACCCE-Research-Report_Factsheet_For-web.pdf

Australian Centre to Counter Child Exploitation. (2025, September 7). *41 per cent jump in online child sexual exploitation reports underscores need for whole-of-community approach.* https://www.accce.gov.au/news-and-media/news/41-cent-jump-online-child-sexual-exploitation-reports-underscores-need-whole-community-approach

Burke, T. (2025, September 4). *Act now, stay secure to protect yourself online.* Department of Home Affairs, Australian Government. https://minister.homeaffairs.gov.au/TonyBurke/Pages/act-now-stay-secure-to-protect-yourself-online.aspx

eSafety Commissioner. (2024). *Levelling up to stay safe: Young people's experiences navigating the joys and risks of online gaming*, Canberra: Australian Government.

eSafety Commissioner. (2024). *Young people and gaming*, Canberra: Australian Government.

1 Being aware of your digital footprint

The piercing ring of the bell echoed through the high school corridors, signalling the end of the first class as students quickly gathered their laptops and rushed to the door, heading to their next class. "Here he is, the man of the hour," an animated Jett yelled as he crossed paths with his friend, Josh, who *lifted his head just enough to make eye contact* but did not seem at all amused with the banter. "What? Are you nervous?" Jett asked. "If you have got cold feet, I'm happy to do it for you, no worries at all," Jett said jokingly. "No, no," Josh responded. "It is not the debate, Jett, it is not the debate. It is not that." "Then what is it?" Jett pressed, "You look crushed, man." "Ah … it is the work experience at DFAT," Josh replied with a deep sigh. "Dad just texted me to say that I did not make it," Josh added. "They made a U-turn on their offer to me." "After they have already agreed to take you?" Jett questioned. "Yep," Josh replied with a heavy heart. "I am really sorry, man," Jett said sympathetically as he put his hand on his friend's shoulder. "Apparently, they did a background check and unearthed an Instagram photo of us drinking at Emily's birthday party last year," Josh explained as he continued to vent his frustration. "I wish I were not tagged in that photo. It isn't fair. I really wanted to work for DFAT in the future. How could I have known that a silly mistake like that could have such a long-lasting effect on me? I am only 17." *Conversation fades out.*

Every action online leaves a trace

Digital identities can significantly influence future opportunities, personal reputations, and online security. In Australia, children begin using the internet at an average age of just under eight years old, contributing to the early development of extensive digital footprints. Research indicates that 80% of children in developed countries already have a digital footprint before the age of two, often as a result of parental sharing, commonly referred to as "sharenting", on social media platforms.

By the time you reach adolescence, your digital presence is often already well established. Nearly 98% of teens report using at least one social media platform

DOI: 10.4324/9781003681731-2

on a regular basis. In Australia, in 2024, Snapchat was used daily by 59% of teens, followed closely by TikTok at 57% and Instagram at 56%. At the same time, many teenagers underestimate just how visible and permanent their online activity can be. Research shows that 92% of teens go online every day, with almost 46% saying they are online almost constantly. While this level of engagement reflects confidence and familiarity with technology, it also means that a digital footprint is being created early and repeatedly. Frequent posting, messaging, searching, and scrolling all contribute to a growing record of personal data that can be collected, shared, analysed, and stored long after the moment feels forgotten.

Teens are worried about how their data is being protected

Despite how active teens are online, many feel uneasy about how digital platforms collect, store, and use their personal information. A significant number worry that their data could be used against them in the future. Around 35% of teens say they have regretted posting something online, and 41% report deleting content because they were worried about how it might affect their reputation. Nearly three-quarters of teens believe that what they post online will follow them into adulthood, a well-founded belief, given that 43% of employers screen candidates' social media profiles during hiring, and one in three university admissions officers report reviewing applicants' online presence as part of the selection process.

In 2022, high school quarterback Marcus Stokes lost a scholarship offer from the University of Florida after a video he posted on social media showed him singing along to a song containing a racial slur. The video went viral, prompting the university to withdraw its offer of a football scholarship. Stokes publicly apologised, saying he regretted his choice of words and accepted the consequences of his actions.

At the same time, many teenagers experience a gap between what they believe and what they do online. Surveys show that most teens care about privacy and want platforms to clearly explain what data is collected, ask permission before sharing it, and give users more control. Yet many also feel powerless, believing they have little influence over how companies track and use their information.

Your online data is regularly accessed and sold

The selling of user data collected through apps is a substantial and rapidly growing sector. This industry encompasses thousands of companies that collect, aggregate, and sell billions of data elements on individuals, often with minimal oversight. For instance, advertising firms reportedly track 2.3 billion people globally, maintain over 7,000 data points on each United States individual, enable highly personalised advertising, but also raise significant privacy concerns. Additionally, a study found that 80% of fitness applications share user data with third parties, including data brokers and advertisers, highlighting the pervasive nature of data sharing across various digital platforms.

Not seeing the immediate effects of doing things online leads to a sense of "it won't happen to me", where you might worry about privacy in theory but still assume nothing bad will happen to you personally, or that data collection is simply the price of being online. This mismatch between awareness and action makes it easier to ignore long-term risks, even as your digital footprint continues to grow, be analysed by AI, and be reused in ways you may never fully see or understand.

Things you do online can affect your future opportunities

The sale of user data means that even minor illegal activities documented online can impact future opportunities. For instance, employers and insurance companies may access this information, potentially leading to negative outcomes such as job application rejections or higher insurance premiums.

A recent New Zealand study revealed that young people's digital footprints can have serious, long-term consequences. The research showed that online interactions contribute to a lasting trail of "digital trace data" collected by social media companies, which can be sold to third parties, including employers and insurance companies. One participant even admitted, "Facebook probably knows I sell drugs," highlighting the level of data surveillance involved, the intensity of tracking of online interactions that occur, and the lack of concern regarding the real-world consequences.

A 17-year-old Louisiana high school student, Kaylee, had her role as student government president revoked and her scholarship support withdrawn after a video showing her twerking at a private homecoming after-party was shared on social media. The principal viewed the clip and decided her behaviour reflected poorly on the school, leading to the loss of leadership and scholarship opportunities, leaving Kaylee feeling devastated and unfairly judged based on a moment captured online.

Your digital footprint can haunt you

Josh's mistake came from the belief that his past online actions wouldn't have lasting consequences. He assumed that being tagged in a post was harmless and didn't consider how publicly accessible content could affect his future. Like many others, he prioritised the enjoyment of online social interactions and the desire to be part of the moment over potential risks. He must have believed that online reputation issues were something that happened to other people, not him. His regret reflects the "privacy paradox", where he valued his privacy but didn't take proactive steps to protect his digital footprint.

The digital world is a complex space where perception and reality often don't align. As a teenager, you might believe you have nothing to hide, that you are not interesting enough to be targeted, or that negative consequences won't happen to you. These assumptions create blind spots in how you manage your digital footprint, leaving you more vulnerable than you realise.

The illusion of control

One of the biggest psychological influences on digital behaviour is the tendency to prioritise immediate rewards over long-term consequences, a phenomenon known as hyperbolic discounting. The instant gratification of likes, shares, and recognition often feels more important than potential risks, like privacy breaches or reputational harm. When choosing between online interactions that offer instant validation and the consideration of the long-term impact of your actions, you are more likely to focus on the present. The need for social approval can overshadow logical assessments of potential dangers, leading to choices that may have lasting consequences.

In reality, the decisions you make when engaging in the following all contribute to a digital footprint that is difficult to erase:

- ☑ Browsing and searching for information online
- ☑ Posting personal photos, videos, or updates
- ☑ Being tagged in photos, videos, or posts shared by others
- ☑ Commenting, liking, or participating in online discussions
- ☑ Using AI tools and the prompts you enter

Another common mistake you can make is believing that online anonymity provides control and protection. Private messages, disappearing posts, and anonymous forums can create the illusion that your actions are temporary and untraceable. But in reality, digital interactions are rarely as private as they seem. Screenshots, data tracking, and algorithms ensure that everything you do online leaves a lasting digital trail and one that can resurface when you least expect it.

> **Even when you delete something online, it does not always disappear completely.** For example, social media platforms often retain copies of deleted posts, messages, or data, meaning your content can still exist long after you think it is gone.

Your online identity is how you are judged offline

The online world offers an unparalleled opportunity for self-expression and identity formation. The desire to belong, connect, and engage with others plays a fundamental role in shaping online behaviour. Social media platforms provide immediate reinforcement through likes, comments, and shares, making digital interactions highly rewarding.

Exposure to content from your online friends can create pressure to share more personal experiences. This pressure is closely linked to the phenomenon of fear of missing out (FOMO), where you feel compelled to participate in online trends, share your location, or document daily activities to remain socially relevant. The result is an expanding digital footprint that reflects a growing archive of personal data, interactions, and behaviours.

Carefully crafting your digital presence to project a desired image is a process strongly influenced by impression management. Every post, comment, and interaction contributes to your digital identity, shaped by both personal aspirations and social expectations. This process encourages you to share content that aligns with your self-image while also influencing your sense of identity.

Why do people act differently online? The anonymity of the internet and a perceived detachment from real-world consequences can lead to the *online disinhibition effect*. In digital spaces, you may behave in ways you would not in face-to-face interactions by expressing opinions more freely or engaging in behaviours you might otherwise avoid. Managing multiple identities across online and offline spaces becomes increasingly difficult, as content intended for one audience can easily be seen by another, leading to unintended consequences for personal relationships and future opportunities.

Example

- *Would Josh have allowed his photo to be posted with his name displayed all over the school?* Likely not, as he would have been aware that teachers, his parents, and other adults could see it and recognise that he was engaging in inappropriate activities.
- *Would he have shown the same photo to a prospective employer?* Certainly not, as it would have reflected poorly on his decision-making and judgement.

It won't happen to me, as I am not important

One major psychological factor shaping your digital behaviour is the third-person effect, which is the belief that online risks are more likely to affect others than yourself. This false sense of invulnerability can lead to riskier online behaviour, as the misuse of personal data often feels like a distant possibility rather than a real threat. As a result, you may overlook privacy settings, overshare personal details, or engage in interactions you would likely avoid in face-to-face settings.

The privacy paradox adds another layer of complexity. Many young people express concerns about online privacy, yet their actions don't always reflect these concerns. This disconnect is often influenced by habitual behaviours and trust heuristics, where you assume digital platforms will protect your data simply because nothing bad has happened to you yet.

You've probably heard stories about people getting into trouble over something they posted online. But you might think ***that won't happen to me. I'm not important.*** It's easy to assume that privacy settings will keep you safe, but they don't offer full protection. Many people underestimate risks like data permanence, surveillance, and third-party access to personal information. Instead of critically evaluating these dangers, it's common to assume everything will be fine. This mindset leads to reactive privacy management, where you only adjust your settings or take precautions after something goes wrong and when it's already too late.

What Josh experienced with DFAT is unfortunately far more common than most teenagers realise. Around the world, there are many examples of young people losing important opportunities because of something they posted online that seemed innocent or was simply meant to be fun. What you share online can shape how others see you, including schools, employers and even future partners. A moment that feels harmless at the time does not always stay in the moment. Once it is posted, it can become part of your permanent digital record and follow you long after the fun has faded.

Check-in: Are you at risk of leaving a digital footprint that could create issues for you?

- ❒ You have posts or photos you wouldn't want a future boss, teacher, or family member to see
- ❒ Your accounts are public, or you accept requests from people you don't really know
- ❒ You share personal details like your school, location, or routine
- ❒ You post or comment without thinking first
- ❒ You've been tagged in things you're not proud of
- ❒ You send things privately that would embarrass you if made public
- ❒ You assume "It won't happen to me" or that deleted posts disappear forever

If you checked **one or more**, you may be leaving behind a digital footprint that could create problems in the future.

If you checked **three or more**, it's time to take action right now to clean up your online presence and reset your habits.

Who tracks your online movements, and what information is collected about you?

Online cookies track what websites you visit

The websites you visit track you. This tracking is facilitated using tiny pieces of text called cookies that these sites store on your machines the first time you visit them. The next time you visit these websites, your browser sends these cookies to these websites. This is how these websites recognise you and personalise your online experience according to your past behaviour.

These websites collect information about you to serve you targeted personalised advertisements. But the tracking goes beyond the websites you visit. The moment you visit these websites, your information travels to other third-party websites with which these websites are affiliated. In addition to the cookies that travel back and forth between your browser and the websites you visit, you can also be tracked using third-party cookies. These third-party cookies travel back and forth between your browser and the websites of the businesses that served you advertisements on the website you visited. That is, a single visit to your daily news site can result in your browser downloading all the cookies associated with the third-party websites on which your daily news site served you advertisements on their behalf.

Applications track everything about you

The apps on your smartphone and device also track you. While cookies are no longer used in this tracking, the apps have built-in tools that make them capable of tracking you and analysing your app usage. Apps can determine your exact location at any point in time using GPS, Wi-Fi, Bluetooth, and cellular antennas. Apps may gain access to your camera and microphone, which can enable them to film you or record your audio without you even being aware.

> **Read more information on protecting yourself from location tracking in** Chapter 2: Smartphone Privacy, Security Settings, and Your Identifying Information

Apps can also gain access to your contacts, calendar, and photos and files on your smartphone. Apps also track how you use them; for example, how often you use the apps, how long you spend on the apps in a single day, what content you view or skip, and which of the apps' features you use more than others. Most of the apps you use are front ends for digital services that require access to backend databases or servers with which you have accounts. As such, the apps not only authenticate you to the backend databases or servers and authorise you to use the digital services available to you, but you also use them to update your account details with the digital services provider. The apps collect your full name, date of birth, email address, physical address, phone number, etc., and transfer this information to a remote server database for processing, access from multiple devices, and backing up.

Search engines track everything you search for

Tracking is also done through a method called digital fingerprinting. This form of tracking takes place not only on the device you are using but across all the other devices you use. This is how the advertisements you see on one device follow you onto your other devices. Search engines also keep a record of all your searches. Whether you searched while you are logged in to your search engine account or while logged out, a record of your search activity is kept by your search engine. In addition, your browser also saves a record of your internet activities on your machine. You can find these records in your Temp folder. If you don't want your computer to remember your search history, use the Incognito mode.

The media have reported on numerous cases in which law enforcement authorities charged potential offenders based on evidence, including search histories, found on their machines. The good news is that you can make it difficult for your search engine to track you. For example, you can stop Google from saving your history. When you click on your Google icon, it will show you if your search history is saved. You can also pause your Google Activity by clicking on Search Personalisation and from there clicking on My Google Activity. Make sure your Web & App Activity, Timeline, and YouTube History are all off.

Social media tracks every interaction

Social media platforms also track all your movements online, even if you don't have an account with them. If you visit a website that contains the social media platform's widgets (tiles), then these widgets act as CCTV cameras silently watching your browsing activities. If you have an account with them and if you browse the internet while logged in to your social media platforms, then the surveillance is accurate because your identity is known to these sites. If you don't have an account with them or browse the internet when you are not logged in to your social media platform, then the surveillance is probabilistic, affecting only your device. But with cross-device tracking and machine learning, this tracking can be made more accurate. However, while you can't stop your social media apps from tracking you, you can stop them from remembering your history.

Each social media app has a way to delete your search history in its app settings. To limit ad personalisation, you can also turn off ads based on your activity, ads using their partner data, and location-based ads. You should also prevent the social media apps from tracking you outside the apps by turning off the "Allow Apps to Request to Track" feature (iPhone) and deleting the advertising ID, and turning off the ad personalisation feature (Android).

Internet service providers (ISP) track all your online activities

Your ISP also keeps a record of all your internet activities. By law, your ISP is required to store the metadata (logs) of your internet activities for five years. Law enforcement authorities can request this metadata if the need arises. Similarly, all your financial transactions in which you used your credit card, debit card, or any other online payment method are recorded by your financial institutions. Financial institutions are obliged to share certain financial information about you with the Taxation Office, Social Services, etc.

How can you minimise your digital footprint?

You can't erase your existing digital footprint or prevent data from being collected about you. But you can minimise the tracking to a great extent.

1 Managing your cookies

Let us first look at web browsing and searching, where your digital footprint often begins. Even private or casual searches can be tracked, stored, and linked back to you over time:

- If you live in Europe, GDPR regulations give you greater control over your data. You can choose to block or limit tracking by denying non-essential cookies on the websites you visit, reducing how your online activity is followed and recorded, including Performance Cookies, Targeting Cookies, Functional Cookies, and especially the Strictly Necessary Cookies.
- If you live outside of Europe, you don't have a choice to reject the Strictly Necessary Cookies from following you. To deny all other types of cookies, such as Performance Cookies, Targeting Cookies, and Functional Cookies, you need to actively manage the cookie settings by selecting which cookies you will allow and which ones you want to reject, which is inconvenient if you only want to visit a website once.

2 Turning on browser blocker extensions

You can also reduce how much you are tracked online by using ad blockers and tracking blockers, which are simple extensions you can add to your web browser. Don't install non-native browser extensions or plugins provided by third parties, as these can track your online activities, or worse, contain malicious code that threat actors, i.e., cyber criminals, can inject into the browser extension to steal your sensitive information, like your logon credentials. You should also make it a habit to always clear the stored cookies and site data. To do this in Firefox, go to Settings > Privacy & Security > Clear Data under Cookies and Site Data. You can set Firefox to delete cookies and site data when it closes.

When it comes to browsing, Google Chrome may not be the best option if you are concerned about your privacy. You can use other browsers, like Firefox, which is known for putting the user's privacy at the forefront. With Firefox, you can adjust the privacy settings according to your privacy needs. For example, you can set up Firefox to "Never Remember History", and you can set it up to block social media trackers, cross-site cookies, crypto miners, and fingerprinters. Similarly, when it comes to searching, Google may not be your best option if you don't want your searches to follow you and don't want to receive search results that Google knows you want to receive. You can use a search engine, like DuckDuckGo or Qwant, which are both known for being privacy-focused and don't track users or store information about them.

3 Use a virtual private network (VPN)

If you want to search anonymously, you can use a VPN or an anonymising tool. If you use a VPN, please note that the VPN will proxy all your information through it, and the VPN provider also gets a copy of your sensitive data. Therefore, if you must use a VPN, it must be from a trusted source. Anonymising tools like TOR can tunnel all your connections through the internet via different hops, hiding your IP address, but the downside is that by using them, you can draw attention to yourself. For example, law enforcement authorities may suspect you are hiding your identity because you must be doing something nefarious.

4 Adjust social media privacy settings

If you are using social media accounts for private purposes, you should consider making your social media accounts private. You should also substantially limit the personal information you share online. You should not share information, like your full name, your complete date of birth, your address, where you were born, your financial transactions, the names of your parents, or your favourite food or your favourite pet. Business entities, like your bank or credit card provider, use the answers to these questions to identify you. Cyber criminals should not have access to these sensitive details about you. You should adjust the privacy settings on all your social media accounts, restricting access to your personal information to only people you know and trust.

Social media platforms now make it possible for you to link your social media accounts with each other for maximum exposure and reach. This, however, raises important privacy and security concerns. From a privacy perspective, linking your accounts can make it possible for anyone to track your social media presence across multiple platforms. Also, if you post anonymously on one platform and use your real identity on another social media platform, anyone can easily connect your anonymous account to the one where you post using your real name. In this regard, it will be hard for you to maintain separate personas on multiple accounts. From a security perspective, if attackers hacked into one of your social media accounts, it would become easier for them to hack into your other linked accounts. Linking your social media accounts, for example, your Facebook, your Instagram, and your WhatsApp, can lead to more targeted advertising, an invasive personalised experience, and increased surveillance because this linking will make it possible for these social media platforms to share your data among each other, especially if they are, like in this case, from the same company, Meta.

5 Ensure good password practices

You should also avoid using the same password for multiple social media accounts. If one social media account is compromised, attackers can use the compromised password with all your other social media accounts. In this regard, you should consider enabling multi-factor authentication (MFA) for your social media accounts for optimal privacy and security. You should also avoid synchronising your social media accounts across multiple devices. This will prevent attackers from accessing your social media accounts via a device you lost, or that was stolen or compromised.

6 Stop using your real name publicly online

You should also avoid posting comments on public forums using your real name or a handle that you use with your other social media accounts. If you must contribute to online public forums, you should use a pseudonym. Please note that if your account in these public forums is compromised or if the public forum platform has been hacked, then your identity can be inferred from your account details, linking you to all your anonymous posts. For this reason, it is best if you don't post anything online that you don't want people to know you said, including your views about race, religion, politics, gender, ethnicity, and sexual orientation.

What to do if your digital footprint has created a problem for you?

Josh is probably feeling a mix of shock, disappointment, and concern for what this means for his future. He might be asking himself how one photo could derail such an important opportunity, especially since he didn't post it himself, and what else could be out there that could create further issues.

Josh can also acknowledge what happened without blaming others. Even if he wasn't the one who posted the photo, he can take responsibility for managing his digital footprint in the future.

1 Start by assessing your digital presence

Before you can fix any problems, you need to understand what information about you is already out there. Assessing your digital presence helps you spot risks early and take informed action to reduce them:

- **Search your name** and key personal details (like your email or usernames) on search engines to see what appears publicly.
- **Review all your social media accounts** and scroll through your posts, photos, comments, likes, and anything you've been tagged in.
- **Check privacy settings** on each platform to see what others can view, especially people who aren't connected to you.
- **Use Google's "Results about You"** tool to find and remove your information from search results, and consider accessing premium tools. Services like **DeleteMe**, **PrivacyBee**, **Mozilla Monitor**, and **Optery** can scan the internet for your personal information and, depending on the subscription level you choose, remove that data on your behalf.

Search online for: "[App name] remove my details from internet"; "[App name] delete my online information"; "Free tool to remove my personal details online"; "Check my leaked data online"

2 Take control and clean up what you can

Your digital footprint is not fixed, and you are not powerless if something online no longer represents who you are. Taking control means reviewing what is already out there and cleaning up what you can to reduce future risks and protect your reputation by:

- **Deleting old posts** or photos that no longer reflect who you are or that could be misunderstood.
- **Untagging yourself** from photos or posts that others have shared if they're not appropriate or you didn't approve of them.
- **Asking friends** to remove content they've shared about you if it could negatively impact your reputation.
- **Updating your privacy settings** across all platforms to restrict who can see your posts, tag you, or access your personal information.

Setting your profile to private is a good start, but it's not enough. If a post could harm your reputation or privacy, it's best to remove it completely. Even with privacy settings in place, there's always a chance you might accept a friend request from someone you think you know, when in reality, they may be trying to gather information about you.

3 Go a step further

Even after cleaning up your accounts and posts, your personal information can still exist online in places you may not control. Taking extra steps can help limit what others can find and protect your digital footprint over the long-term:

- Turn off data collection and sharing on apps and platforms.
- Delete old accounts or apps you no longer need, as they may still hold your personal data.
- If damaging content appears in search engine results that you can't remove yourself, consider requesting removal directly from the platform or the search engine provider. Some search engines have tools to remove outdated or harmful content.

4 Actively manage your online identity and data

Your digital footprint can be a powerful tool when used intentionally. By actively shaping your online presence, you have the opportunity to build a positive digital identity that supports your future goals.

Think of your digital footprint as part of your *personal brand*. Every post, photo, and interaction is how you are perceived by others. Before sharing content or allowing data about your actions to be collected, pause and ask yourself:

"Would I be comfortable if a future boss, teacher, partner, or family member saw I was doing this?" If the answer is "no" or even "maybe", it's worth reconsidering.

Make sure any online information or profiles highlight:

- Your interests, values, and aspirations
- Academic or sport achievements, community involvement, and volunteer experiences
- Content that reflects well on you would be positively viewed by future employers, educators, or anyone in your personal life

If sharing certain information about yourself wouldn't be acceptable to everybody you know now or might meet in the future, think twice before doing it online.

5 Take responsibility for your actions

It is important that if your online actions have caused issues, you should take responsibility. Avoid blame shifting or downplaying what has happened. Acknowledge the impact and take active steps to repair the harm that has been done, whether that means having a conversation with someone affected or apologising for your actions.

If Josh still wants to pursue a career at DFAT or a similar organisation, he might consider writing a letter explaining what he learned from this experience. Showing maturity and growth can sometimes turn a setback into a second chance.

Conclusion

This chapter focuses on how you can manage your digital footprint when searching the web, browsing the internet, using social media, and accessing online services. In Europe, users have the right to be forgotten. Elsewhere, nothing is forgotten. Anything you do online leaves a digital trace that can last for years, and sometimes forever. What feels insignificant now can later influence opportunities and experiences that matter most to you in the future. The fact that you don't see it in Google search results does not mean it is not there. For this reason, you must be fully equipped with the skills to minimise the tracking. If you think you are not important, then ask yourself: why are companies spending billions of dollars to find out everything about you? If you think that because you have nothing to hide, you have nothing to worry about, it is not about having something to hide; it is about having something to protect. Something that is no one else's business to know about. The key thing is control. You are entitled to control who knows what about you. If you don't exercise this control over your online presence, your online presence will control your entire life for you without you even knowing.

Key terms

- Digital footprint
- Sharenting
- Privacy paradox
- Hyperbolic discounting
- Online anonymity
- Online disinhibition effect
- Impression management
- Third-person effect
- Data permanence
- Reactive privacy management
- Data tracking
- Algorithms
- Cookies
- GPS
- ISP
- VPN
- IP address
- Digital fingerprinting

Bibliography

Bartholomew, K. (2017, June 28). *Snapchat's Snap Map feature raises safety concerns*. ABC News. https://www.abc.net.au/news/2017-06-28/snapchats-snap-map-feature-raises-safety-concern/8660066

Bessant, C. (2017, September 20). *Too much information? More than 80% of children have an online presence by the age of two*. The Conversation. https://theconversation.com/too-much-information-more-than-80-of-children-have-an-online-presence-by-the-age-of-two-83251

Booth, G. (2024, September 3). *Social media negatively impacting teens' life satisfaction*. Australian National University. https://www.anu.edu.au/news/all-news/social-media-negatively-impacting-teens-life-satisfaction

Chantiri, L. (2025, October 16). *Gen Z in the firing line as employers scrutinise social media posts.* The Sydney Morning Herald. https://www.smh.com.au/business/workplace/gen-z-in-the-firing-line-as-employers-scrutinise-social-media-posts-20251016-p5n32n.html

Delaney, A. (2023, July 13). *Woman's warning over Snapchat Snap Maps feature after terrifying encounter.* 7NEWS. https://7news.com.au/technology/snapchat/womans-warning-over-snapchat-snap-maps-feature-after-terrifying-encounter--c-11265262

Elgersma, M. (2017, July 2). *Why Snapchat's Snap Map should concern parents.* CNN. https://edition.cnn.com/2017/07/02/opinions/snap-map-privacy-opinion-elgersma/index.html

Faverio, M., & Sidoti, O. (2024, December 12). *Teens, social media and technology 2024.* Pew Research Center. https://www.pewresearch.org/internet/2024/12/12/teens-social-media-and-technology-2024/

GBG. (2022, March 11). *One in seven smartphone users say they have been a victim of identity fraud in the past year.* https://www.gbg.com/en/news/one-in-seven-smartphone-users-say-they-have-been-a-victim-of-identity-fraud-in-the-past-year/

Help Net Security. (2022, March 11). *Young adults hit hardest by identity fraud.* https://www.helpnetsecurity.com/2022/03/11/smartphone-users-identity-fraud/

Howarth, J. (2024). *Identity theft statistics and trends.* Exploding Topics. https://explodingtopics.com/blog/identity-theft-stats

Ironmonger, L. (2024, September 2). *'It gave me the ick': When friendly surveillance crosses the line.* The Sydney Morning Herald. https://www.smh.com.au/lifestyle/life-and-relationships/it-gave-me-the-ick-when-friendly-surveillance-crosses-the-line-20240731-p5jy49.html

Jackson, B. (2025, January 9). *Fitness apps sucking up 21 different types of user data, study finds.* News.com.au. https://www.news.com.au/technology/fitness-apps-sucking-up-21-different-types-of-user-data-study-finds/news-story/aaed2d7eee252536c90369aa917fd156

Kaplan. (2024, January 30). *Kaplan survey: College admissions officers think it's OK to visit applicants' social media, but most don't.* https://kaplan.com/about/press-media/kaplan-survey-college-admissions officers applicant-social-media

Luthi, B. (2025, May 30). *U.S. fraud and identity theft losses topped $12.7 billion in 2024.* Experian. https://www.experian.com/blogs/ask-experian/identity-theft-statistics/

Madden, M., Lenhart, A., Cortesi, S., Gasser, U., Duggan, M., Smith, A., & Beaton, M. (2013, May 21). *Teens, social media, and privacy.* Pew Research Center. https://assets.pewresearch.org/wp-content/uploads/sites/14/2013/05/PIP_TeensSocialMediaandPrivacy_PDF.pdf

Pandey, M. (2023, October 4). *US high school student loses scholarship over social media twerking video.* NDTV. https://www.ndtv.com/offbeat/us-high-school-student-loses-scholarship-over-social-media-twerking-video-4459999

Psychology Society of Australia. (2024). *Australian teens trapped by social media apps as they struggle to disconnect.* https://psychology.org.au/about-us/news-and-media/aps-in-the-media/2024/australian-teens-trapped-by-social-media-apps-as-t

The Week. (2018). *Teen tracking app leaks thousands of user passwords.* The Week. https://theweek.com/93739/teen-tracking-app-leaks-thousands-of-user-passwords

Todd, F. (2025, February 4). *Teen mental health app sent kids' data straight to TikTok.* Gizmodo. https://gizmodo.com/teen-mental-health-app-sent-kids-data-straight-to-tiktok-2000557615 van der Sanden, R., Wilkins, C., Rychert, M., & Barratt, M. (2024, May 22). *Facebook probably knows I sell drugs: How young people's digital footprints can threaten their future prospects.* The Conversation.

Yahoo Sports. (2023, January 27). *Nease QB Marcus Stokes dropped after social media video resurfaces.* https://sports.yahoo.com/nease-qb-marcus-stokes-dropped-210428454.html

YouGov. (2024). *Online communication in Australia Survey – Summer 2024* [Data tables]. Snap Inc. YouGov Data Tables Document

2 Smartphone settings and your identifying information

> Encountering the same people in your daily walk can be heart-warming. The comforting feeling is similar to that you experience in a library with a group of strangers – a silent warmth of human connection, free of the burden that comes with having to maintain relationships. But for Melanie, a 17-year-old student who used to enjoy taking her dog for a walk after school, one encounter in the park has shaken her to the core. The first time she saw a man suspiciously staring at her, as he passed her by, she did not make much of it. However, when he turned back the next day as she passed him, she got an eerie feeling. The next day, she decided to go for her walk later than usual in the hope that she would escape him. But he was there, and this time when he saw her, he slowed down and smiled. Melanie instantly picked up her phone and pretended to be talking to her dad. The moment had passed, but spotting him in the shopping mall the following day when she was with her mum grocery shopping, left Melanie petrified. When Melanie's mum confronted him, he pretended to be paralysed with shock, made an excuse to leave and immediately disappeared. Melanie has never encountered this man again on her walks, but the experience made her wonder how he was able to determine her precise whereabouts every time!

Your privacy is more at risk than ever before

In today's digital age, protecting personal information is more important than ever. Adolescents are increasingly worried about their physical safety, especially the unintended exposure of their location and daily routines. In 2022, approximately 1.7 million US children fell victim to data breaches, meaning one in every 43 children had their personal information exposed or compromised.

DOI: 10.4324/9781003681731-3

Personal information versus sensitive information

- *Personal information* is information that can identify you to others as a specific individual. It includes your name, address, phone number, and date of birth.
- *Sensitive information* relates to other private information about you, such as racial origin, religious beliefs, health information, and sexual orientation.

Recent research indicates that many teenagers are unaware of the extent to which their smartphone usage can lead to privacy leaks. In Australia, a 2023 survey revealed that 91% of young people aged 14–17 own a smartphone. However, a significant number of these teens do not take adequate measures to secure their devices.

Thinking it won't happen to you puts you at risk

Globally, concerns over data privacy are escalating among teenagers. A study highlighted that 67% of teenagers in Latin America aged 13–18 express concern about their privacy. Despite these concerns, there remains a substantial gap between awareness and action. A study in the United States found that while 82% of youth claim they don't share personal information online, half don't use privacy settings, and 25% admit they don't know how to use these settings. This phenomenon, where adolescents recognise the risks associated with smartphone use but fail to implement protective measures, is referred to as the "privacy paradox". It underscores the necessity for enhanced education and resources to empower teens to manage their smartphone privacy settings effectively.

A terrifying news story outlined the dangers when a young woman became the target of an attempted kidnapping. The attacker used Snapchat's live location-sharing feature to track her. The kidnapper confronted the victim at gunpoint in a parked car, attempted to pull her out, and caused bruising and temporary hearing loss. He was later sentenced to ten years in prison. Investigators noted that he had added the victim on Snapchat a year earlier and likely located her using the app's live location.

Smartphones are the riskiest devices

Smartphone ownership among teenagers further amplifies privacy risks. Research has shown that 91% of children aged 14–17 own a smartphone, increasing their exposure to data breaches and online threats. Many engage in risky online behaviours or have negative digital experiences, yet 78% mistakenly believe their devices provide complete security. Frequent smartphone use for social media, gaming, and communication often leads children to overlook essential privacy settings that prevent personal data leakage. A lack of awareness about settings such as Bluetooth, Wi-Fi, smartphone naming, and Location Services further increases vulnerability to data exposure. Misconfigured privacy settings can reveal sensitive details, including personal identities and locations.

A study carried out in Australia revealed that 59% of the surveyed teenage participants keep their Location Services ON all the time. This study also revealed that 38% connect to public Wi-Fis and 58% leave their Bluetooth setting ON regularly. Young adolescent survey respondents indicated that they don't take an active approach to checking which apps have access to their microphone or camera. Leaving these settings ON can result in your smartphone, unbeknownst to you, leaking your sensitive information while your phone is in your pocket, while you sleep, or while it is charging.

The outcomes of information loss are severe

In May 2025, the Australian eSafety Commission released research showing that location-sharing apps, including features like Snapchat's Snap Map, are linked to a higher risk of tech-based coercive control, where someone uses digital tracking to monitor or manipulate a partner, normalising constant monitoring instead of respecting privacy. This concern was highlighted in part by the 2023 murder of 21-year-old Lilie James, whose killer tracked her location through Snapchat's map feature, a misuse of smartphone privacy settings that foreshadowed escalating control and contributed to a fatal outcome.

The risks of identifying information leakage extend beyond location privacy risks. Identity theft among young Australians has surged, with reports showing a 31% increase in cases. Many victims unknowingly expose personal information through unsecured smartphones, making them prime targets for cyber criminals and predators.

The risks of identifying information leakage extend well beyond location tracking and are a growing global concern. In the United States, identity theft and fraud have risen sharply, with over 1.1 million identity theft reports and 2.6 million fraud complaints recorded in 2024, resulting in losses of more than $12.7 billion. Younger people are particularly vulnerable, as research shows that younger people experience higher rates of identity fraud than older age groups, largely due to frequent smartphone and social media use. Globally, surveys indicate that around one in seven smartphone users has been a victim of identity fraud, highlighting how unsecured devices, app permissions, and oversharing of personal details can expose individuals to cyber criminals. These trends demonstrate that smartphones often act as a gateway to personal data, making young people prime targets for identity theft, impersonation, and financial exploitation when privacy settings are poorly managed.

Social engineering and online safety

It turned out the man was able to determine Melanie's precise whereabouts every time by checking her location on Snap Map. But how did the man obtain access to this sensitive information? The answer is that he used social engineering.

Social engineering is a psychological manipulation tactic that tricks people into revealing personal details, often without realising it. Predators use social engineering to track victims, access sensitive smartphone data, and exploit personal information. They don't need advanced hacking tools; manipulating trust, impulsive behaviour, and digital habits are often enough. Melanie didn't even realise that she was being targeted. Everything felt and seemed normal. Social engineering is extremely hard to spot before it is too late.

Gathering data from multiple sources

Many teenagers believe, "It won't happen to me," which makes them underestimate personal risk. People assume that if they don't directly share personal information, they're safe, but predators don't need a single source to track someone. Instead, they piece together details from multiple platforms.

What are some examples of how smartphones can share sensitive details about you?

— Public social media posts – especially those with location tags
— Comments or interactions on messaging apps – conversations that reveal habits, routines, or places
— Location information shared in apps – maps, check-ins, or live location features
— Smartphone or Bluetooth device names – can leak real names or identifying details
— Accessing public Wi-Fi networks – can expose location and device information
— Publicly visible AI prompts or shared chat histories – may reveal personal details, interests, routines, or sensitive information if not set to private

Even when you try to be careful, small bits of data can add up. Predators create a full picture of a victim's regular habits simply by connecting the dots. Even if you are cautious in direct conversations, predators can cross-reference details from information shared in apps, tagged locations, smartphone names, and where they connect to public Wi-Fis to piece together their daily routines, frequented places, and social circles.

The illusion of safety: the disinhibition effect

The online disinhibition effect makes people feel safer and more open in digital spaces, including smartphone apps, than in face-to-face interactions. This false sense of security leads adolescents to:

- ☑ Overshare personal details like locations, routines, or plans for the future
- ☑ Trust online "friends" too quickly
- ☑ Engage in conversations they wouldn't have offline
- ☑ Connect with others through Bluetooth, Wi-Fi, or location-sharing services

Predators leverage this by engaging you in casual conversations that gradually extract useful data or connecting to your smartphone when they are near you. Predators exploit this comfort by posing as someone relatable, such as another teen, a trusted adult, or even an influencer. They mimic interests, use casual language, and build familiarity to create trust.

> **What is a "pretext"?** Attackers, including predators, often proceed in accordance with a pretext that they developed to execute the attack. A pretext is the story they tell or the excuse they give their targets to get them to do something, such as accepting their friend's request.

One dangerous tactic is the reciprocity principle, where predators disclose seemingly personal information first. This makes the teen feel obligated to reciprocate by sharing their own details.

> **Example**: A predator might say, "I go to Rivervale High School – where do you go?" This casual exchange feels harmless, but it instantly gives away critical personal information.

Over time, predators use psychological grooming techniques to desensitise you to sharing sensitive information. They start with harmless topics and progressively normalise the sharing of personal or private details, ensuring that the victim remains unaware of the manipulation.

Manipulating social validation needs

Adolescents are highly influenced by social validation, especially when seeking likes, followers, and approval online. Predators exploit this by posing as popular figures or by offering praise and engagement, making you more likely to share personal details to maintain the interaction.

Adolescents' developing brains make them more prone to impulsive behaviour and prioritising short-term rewards over long-term risks. Their strong need for social validation can push them to share personal information, engage in risky location sharing, or accept friend requests or messages from strangers. The privacy paradox, where teens express concern about privacy but fail to take protective measures, further increases their susceptibility.

Predators using social engineering create urgency or fear to pressure you into acting impulsively. This includes urgent friend requests or fabricated emergencies that trick the victim into revealing location information or personal information. Adolescents with underdeveloped impulse control are especially vulnerable to these tactics.

If we revisit Melanie's situation, we can see that, understanding social engineering, she loved sharing moments of her life on Snapchat by checking in at her favourite cafés, posting selfies at school events, and chatting with new online friends. Her account was private, and she thought she was secure. One day, she had a new friend request. She was careful and messaged them asking how they knew each other. The person claimed to be a mutual female friend and said they had met her at a party she had checked into online. They mentioned details from that event, including a discussion about attending different schools but taking similar classes.

She accepted the request as it seemed genuine, even though she didn't quite remember meeting them. Their profile looked real and showed mutual friends, and as they messaged regularly over time, Melanie felt comfortable sharing more about her daily routine. In reality, the person was an older man using deception to gain her trust. What Melanie didn't realise was that her Snap Map was turned ON, allowing him to see her exact location. Every time she went to the gym, school, took her dog for a walk, or went to her best friend's house, he could track her movements in real time.

Check-in: Are you at risk of having your privacy or personal information leaked through your smartphone?

Phone & Settings

- ❒ Your phone name includes your real name.
- ❒ You haven't checked your privacy settings in a long time.

Location & Photos

- ❒ You leave location on for most apps.
- ❒ You've posted photos or stories that show where you live, go to school, or hang out.

Social Media

- ❐ Your accounts are public.
- ❐ You accept or talk to people you don't know offline.

Passwords & Apps

- ❐ You reuse the same password in lots of places.
- ❐ You don't know which apps can access your camera, mic, location, or contacts.

If you checked **one or more**, you are at risk of your personal information being leaked and used against you.

If you checked **three or more**, you need to act quickly to ensure you resolve the major privacy and personal risks you could face.

How does your smartphone leak your identifying information?

Snap Map allows others to track your location

Snapchat introduced Snap Map in 2017. The feature enables users to locate their Snapchat friends on a map if these friends share their locations. The map can show the friends' locations accurately, allowing users to track their Snapchat friends' physical movements with precision. Snap Map can be accessed from within the Snapchat app by tapping the location icon in the bottom-left corner of the screen. The Snapchat friends appear on the map as static Bitmoji avatars, which they have chosen in Snapchat to represent their identities and personas. The friends' Bitmoji avatars appear on the map as giants standing on the buildings in which they are staying.

Under each Bitmoji avatar, the name of the friend, the time they were last seen at that specific location, and the current battery level are displayed. The suburb where the building is located appears at the top of the screen. The map can be displayed in standard format with Bitmoji avatars indicating friends' locations or in satellite view with real-world imagery. In Zoom Out view, friends appear on the map as giants standing on a heat map. Users can Zoom In by pinching the map with two fingers. One of Snap Map's cool features is the Nearby feature, which users can access using the search function in the top-left corner of the screen. The functionality allows users to discover friends within close range. That is, the friends who are currently present in a nearby location. This affordance is designed to encourage face-to-face interaction by making it easy for friends to find each other in person. In addition, Snapchat can send users notifications when there is a Snap Map activity.

Apps can share your location data

Location data can be extremely valuable to predators. In addition to revealing a person's whereabouts at a specific point in time, location data can also tell predators something about who the person is, what they do, and what they enjoy. Predators can use location data to discover patterns about a person's movements over time, enabling them to create an accurate profile of this person. Snap Map is not the only app that can disclose a user's location. There are numerous other apps that can gain access to a user's Location Services and share this information with others, including predators.

Wi-Fi can leak your personal information

Location can also be determined through the Wi-Fi settings. If the Wi-Fi setting on a smartphone is turned ON, the smartphone can leak its location without the smartphone owner even knowing. When a smartphone connects to a Wi-Fi network, it saves the Wi-Fi network name (SSID) and password for future use. When the user comes back within this Wi-Fi's range in the future, the phone sends a probe to this network to try to reconnect, revealing your location. The Wi-Fi sensor also probes all the Wi-Fi antennas the smartphone passes by, even if your Wi-Fi setting is turned OFF. Your journey to school in the morning can be fully reconstructed from this information, and the route you took to travel to school can be accurately plotted on a Google map.

Bluetooth sensors can detect your location

The Bluetooth sensor is perhaps the most dangerous setting to leave ON all the time. The Bluetooth name is the same as your smartphone's name. So, if you wrote your first and last names on your phone "About" tab, then your Bluetooth uses this information to identify your phone to other Bluetooth devices. Studies have shown that a Bluetooth sensor, such as the M5Stack Core 2 ESP32, can detect your smartphone's identifying information, including your full name, location, and even your MAC address. Of course, you need to keep the Bluetooth setting ON so you can connect your smartphone to your AirPods and your CarPlay, etc. But it is important to know that leaving your Bluetooth sensor ON all the time can make your smartphone discoverable to nearby predators, who can track you, or worse, connect to your device or intercept your communication with another device to which you are connected via Bluetooth. This attack is called a man-in-the-middle attack.

The microphone and camera can be accessed by others

The apps that have gained access to your microphone or camera, or that you have given access to, can invade your privacy. Apps that have access to your microphone can listen to your conversations at times, even when you are not using the microphone. While it makes sense for your WhatsApp to have access to your microphone, it makes no sense for your QR Code Scanner app to have access to your microphone. Why does your flashlight app have access to your camera? It does not need to have access to your camera to do its job.

Apps sell your personal information to third-party marketers without you even knowing. For example, they sell your location (GPS) for targeted ads and store promotions and sell your audio recordings to serve you targeted ads about the things you are currently thinking about.

How can you secure your smartphone?

You can secure your smartphone by taking an active approach to managing your smartphone settings, especially with respect to location, Wi-Fi, Bluetooth, microphone, and camera.

1 Manage location settings

Beginning with location, check your smartphone to see which apps have access to your Location Services. On an iPhone, for example, you can do this by going into Settings > Privacy & Security > Location Services. Clicking on Location Services will list all the apps that have gained access to or have been given access to your location. When Location Services is activated, a small arrow in the top-right corner of the smartphone screen, next to the battery recharge indicator, turns blue inside a little circle. Returning to Snap Map, you can hide your location in Snap Map by enabling Ghost Mode, which you can turn on or off from the settings wheel at the top of the Snap Map screen.

2 Secure Wi-Fi and Bluetooth settings

To view all the Wi-Fi networks that your iPhone, for example, remembers, go to Wi-Fi settings and click on Edit at the top-right corner of your screen. You will find all the Wi-Fi networks that your iPhone remembers listed below. Delete them, except, of course, for your home Wi-Fi network and your school or work networks. Do the same with your Bluetooth. Go to your Bluetooth settings and take note of the devices that have synced or paired with your device. If you don't recognise any device, remove it.

3 Lock down your microphone and camera settings

You should also always keep an eye on which apps have access to your microphone and camera. Go to your Privacy & Security settings, open your microphone app, and observe which apps have access to your microphone. When your microphone is activated, a tiny filled dot appears at the top right of your smartphone screen, next to your battery recharge indicator, usually in orange or green. Repeat this process with your camera. Check which apps can turn ON your camera at times without you knowing you are being filmed. When your camera is activated, a tiny filled green dot appears at the top right of your smartphone screen, next to your battery recharge indicator.

4 Secure your Contacts

You should also check to see which apps have access to your Contacts. The most common apps that often request access to your Contacts are Phone/Messages/FaceTime,Mail/Gmail/Outlook/Meet/Messenger, Facebook/Instagram/Snapchat/TikTok. On an iPhone, you do this by going to Settings > Privacy & Security > Contacts. While none of these apps can access your Contacts without your knowledge or permission, sometimes a user grants access to these apps by accident, like tapping Allow instead of Deny. This is why it is worth double-checking which apps have access to your Contacts. One more thing: check that your smartphone is not managed using a Mobile Device Management (MDM) system, which is used by companies, schools, or organisations to manage smartphones remotely. In Android, it is called Android Enterprise. You can verify if your iPhone is being managed remotely by going to Settings > General > VPN and Device Management. If nothing is listed there, then your phone is not under MDM.

5 Check your other key smartphone privacy settings

Here are four steps you can take to secure your smartphone.

[1] Use the Safety Check feature in your iPhone (with iOS 16 or later) to review and manage your privacy settings. You can access the Safety Check feature in your iPhone by going to Settings > Privacy & Security > Safety Check.

If you are an Android user, the Privacy Dashboard[1] will enable you to see which apps have access to your Camera, Microphone, and Location. To access Privacy Dashboard, go to Settings > Privacy & Security > Privacy. To change app permissions, go to Settings > Apps, tap the app you want to change permissions for, and select Permissions.

By clicking on Manage Sharing & Access, you can remove access on an app-by-app basis. The same goes with people. You can select a person and then remove their access to your iPhone. For example, you can remove their access to your Find My feature. For more information on this feature, visit https://apple.co/safety. If your iPhone's security has been compromised or your personal safety is at risk, you can use the Emergency Reset feature in Safety Check to immediately remove access for all people and all apps. Always back up your data before pressing any reset button.

[2] Switch off services that you don't use. If you are not using a specific service on your phone, turn it off. If you are not using map apps or any other apps that require Location Services, then turn off Location Services. While doing so will not completely stop the tracking of your location, it will, to a great extent, limit it. The same goes for your Wi-Fi and Bluetooth services. If you are not using them, you should turn them off.

[3] Anonymise your device, or what the cybersecurity experts call "hiding the device". It is understandably inconvenient to leave the Bluetooth service off all the time, because, as mentioned above, you may want to connect your AirPods to your phone. Therefore, if you can't switch off the above services, you can at least de-identify your phone by replacing your real name on your phone with something else with which your parents, caregivers, and friends can associate.

Back to Melanie's situation, instead of using "Melanie Smith's iPhone7", use something like "Dog Walker". This will prevent predators from linking your phone's data to you. By removing the reference to iPhone7, you are also not giving away the type of phone you are using. This will prevent predators from linking your phone to the security vulnerabilities it is associated with.

[4] Take active control of your smartphone settings. This means going into Settings > Privacy & Security and checking each app's settings and removing access to services from apps that should not have access. You can also now find out which apps have access to which services (Location, Camera, Microphone, Contacts) from the Apps feature, which you can locate from General settings at the bottom of your screen.

What should you do if your sensitive information has been compromised?

For 17-year-old Melanie, realising her privacy had been invaded was overwhelming. But taking the right steps helped her regain control and protect herself in the future. If you ever find yourself in a similar situation, taking immediate action can help prevent further harm.

1 Identify the impact

Before you act, you need to understand exactly what might have been exposed. Ask yourself whether your location has been tracked in real time:

- This includes apps showing where you are, someone knowing where you've been, or notifications revealing your movements.
- Has personal information been accessed or shared without your permission?
- This could be photos, your real name, your phone number, your school, or apps that had camera or microphone access you didn't approve.

- Have you received suspicious messages or contact from someone you don't truly know? Especially if the messages feel pushy, creepy, or ask for more information about you.

Once you understand what type of information was exposed, you can decide what needs to be secured first in relation to your accounts, your phone, your location settings, or your safety offline.

> **Tip**: Check for unusual location activity, unexpected app permissions, or messages from unknown people.

2 Document everything

If someone has stalked, threatened, impersonated, or harassed you, keep detailed records. Documentation protects you and strengthens your case if you need help.

- Take screenshots of texts, DMs, friend requests, profiles, or any suspicious activity.
- Save dates, times, usernames, and platform names.
- Keep notes on any apps or public Wi-Fi you used when the issue happened.
- Record places where your location may have leaked, like stories, check-ins, or photos.

This documentation helps adults, police, schools, or online platforms understand what happened and act quickly.

3 Block and report the behaviour

If someone has harassed you, impersonated you, tracked your location, or accessed your account:

- Block the person immediately. Blocking stops them from contacting you or viewing your profile.
- Report the account or behaviour to the platform.
- Almost every application, including Instagram, Snapchat, TikTok, Discord, and gaming platforms, lets you report threats, impersonation, stalking, or inappropriate messages.
- If someone created a fake account pretending to be you, report it as impersonation so the platform can remove it.

Blocking and reporting are important not only for your safety, but also to stop the offender from targeting others.

> **Search online for**: "[App name] how to report harassment"; "[App name] block or report user"; "[App name] privacy settings location sharing"

4 Monitor for further threats

Even after the immediate attack, stay alert:

- Keep an eye out for new accounts that might be the same person using a different name.
- Be more cautious with friend requests, even if the profile looks "normal".
- Don't click on unexpected links, QR codes, or files sent by strangers.
- If your location was exposed, avoid going alone to places where the person might expect you to be, and bring a friend or trusted adult.
- Turn off location sharing for apps that don't need it.
- Think of this stage as tightening the locks and watching for anyone who tries to get back in.

5 Seek legal or professional help if necessary

If you feel unsafe or if someone continues to contact you:

- Tell a trusted adult, such as a parent, teacher, school counsellor, or guardian.
- Report stalking, threats, or harassment to local police. They take cyber harassment and cyberstalking seriously.
- Use government online safety agencies or cyber crime reporting websites for guidance and next steps.
- If passwords or accounts were compromised, get help from a professional or your phone provider to secure your device.

You are never expected to handle serious online harm alone. Getting help early prevents the situation from escalating.

Legal tip: Report to police if someone uses your smartphone privacy leakage to stalk, threaten, harass, impersonate you, access your personal information without permission, or coerce you. These actions are highly illegal.

Search online for "[Your country] Report Cyber Threats"; "[Your country] Online Safety Reports"; "Teen Helpline [Your country]"

Conclusion

This chapter focused on the leakage of your identifying information from your smartphone without your knowledge. This form of leakage is dangerous not only because it is unintentional but also because it is stealthy. It can make you vulnerable to attacks, such as the social engineering attack that Melanie survived. For this reason, it is important that you are fully aware of how to manage your smartphone's privacy and security settings. There are four steps that you can take to secure your smartphone: [1] review and manage your privacy settings, [2] switch off services you are not using and if you can't, [3] hide the identity of your phone, and the best step is for you to [4] take active control of your smartphone privacy and security settings. By actively adjusting each app's access to your services, you will limit information leakage from your phone, keeping it secure. This chapter also offers you steps on what to do if your sensitive information has been compromised.

Key terms

- Online data
- Personal information
- Privacy paradox
- Social engineering
- Online disinhibition
- Social validation
- MAC address
- SSID
- BSSID
- Sensor
- Avatar
- Pretext

Note

1 https://www.android.com/intl/en_au/safety/privacy/#safety-privacy-dashboard.

Bibliography

Al-Saggaf, Y., & Maclean, J. (2024). *Protecting children from smartphone's leakage of security sensitive information* [Final report]. eSafety Commissioner Online Safety Grants Program; Charles Sturt University.

Android. (n.d.). *Safety & privacy*. https://www.android.com/intl/en_au/safety/privacy/#safety-privacy-dashboard

Australian Psychological Society. (2024, May 20). *Australian teens trapped by social media apps as their mental health declines*. https://psychology.org.au/about-us/news-and-media/aps-in-the-media/2024/australian-teens-trapped-by-social-media-apps-as-t

Australian Signals Directorate. (2026, April 9). *Social engineering*. Australian Cyber Security Centre. https://www.cyber.gov.au/threats/types-threats/social-engineering

Bartholomew, K. (2017, June 28). *Snapchat's Snap Map feature raises safety concern*. Australian Broadcasting Corporation. https://www.abc.net.au/news/2017-06-28/snapchats-snap-map-feature-raises-safety-concern/8660066

Delaney, A. (2023, July 13). *Woman's warning over Snapchat Snap Maps feature after terrifying encounter.* 7NEWS. https://7news.com.au/technology/snapchat/womans-warning-over-snapchat-snap-maps-feature-after-terrifying-encounter--c-11265262

Elgersma, C. (2017, July 2). *Snap Map privacy opinion.* CNN. https://edition.cnn.com/2017/07/02/opinions/snap-map-privacy-opinion-elgersma/index.html

eSafety Commissioner. (2025, May 15). *Youth support for tracking apps raises red flag for coercive control.* https://www.esafety.gov.au/newsroom/media-releases/youth-support-for-tracking-apps-raises-red-flag-for-coercive-control

Feathers, T. (2025, February 4). *Teen mental health app sent kids' data straight to TikTok.* Gizmodo. https://gizmodo.com/teen-mental-health-app-sent-kids-data-straight-to-tiktok-2000557615

Federal Trade Commission. (2025, March 10). *New FTC data show a big jump in reported losses to fraud to $12.5 billion in 2024.* https://www.ftc.gov/news-events/news/press-releases/2025/03/new-ftc-data-show-big-jump-reported-losses-fraud-125-billion-2024

GBG. (2023, June 20). *One in seven smartphone users say they have been a victim of identity fraud in the past year.* https://www.gbg.com/en/news/one-in-seven-smartphone-users-say-they-have-been-a-victim-of-identity-fraud-in-the-past-year/

Ghai, S., Magis-Weinberg, L., Stoilova, M., Livingstone, S., & Orben, A. (2022). Social media and adolescent well-being in the Global South. *Current Opinion in Psychology, 46*, 101318. https://doi.org/10.1016/j.copsyc.2022.101318

Goldberg, T. (Kitten). (2022, October 26). *Child identity fraud: The perils of too many screens and social media* [White paper]. https://javelinstrategy.com/whitepapers/child-identity-fraud-perils-too-many-screens-and-social-media

Help Net Security. (2022, March 11). *Young adults hit hardest by identity fraud.* https://www.helpnetsecurity.com/2022/03/11/smartphone-users-identity-fraud/

Hoffman, C. (2019, October 21). *Snapchat's location feature used in several Arizona crimes.* Arizona Republic. https://www.azcentral.com/story/money/business/tech/2019/10/21/snapchat-location-feature-snap-map-used-in-several-arizona-crimes/4045867002/

Howarth, B. (2023, December 5). *Identity theft statistics and trends.* Exploding Topics. https://explodingtopics.com/blog/identity-theft-stats

Ironmonger, L. (2024, July 31). *"It gave me the ick": When friendly surveillance crosses the line.* https://www.smh.com.au/lifestyle/life-and-relationships/it-gave-me-the-ick-when-friendly-surveillance-crosses-the-line-20240731-p5jy49.html

Levy, A. (2025, May 15). *Location-sharing apps linked to increased risk of digital coercive control, eSafety Commission research finds.* https://www.abc.net.au/news/2025-05-15/location-sharing-apps-esafety-commission-coercive-control/105289994

Luthi, B. (2025, May 30). *Identity theft statistics.* Experian. https://www.experian.com/blogs/ask-experian/identity-theft-statistics/

Madden, M., Lenhart, A., Cortesi, S., Gasser, U., Duggan, M., Smith, A., & Beaton, M. (2013, May 21). *Teens, social media, and privacy.* Pew Research Center. https://www.pewresearch.org/internet/2013/05/21/teens-social-media-and-privacy/

Madden, M., Lenhart, A., Cortesi, S., Gasser, U., Duggan, M., Smith, A., & Beaton, M. (2013, May 21). *Part 2: Information sharing, friending, and privacy settings on social media.* In *Teens, social media, and privacy.* Pew Research Center. https://www.pewresearch.org/internet/2013/05/21/part-2-information-sharing-friending-and-privacy-settings-on-social-media/

Office of the Australian Information Commissioner. (n.d.). *What is personal information?* https://www.oaic.gov.au/privacy/your-privacy-rights/your-personal-information/what-is-personal-information

Roberts, M. (2025, November 29). *NSW Lilie James murder location sharing DV tech abuse.* ABC News. https://www.abc.net.au/news/2025-11-29/nsw-lilie-james-murder-location-sharing-dv-tech-abuse/106072984

The Week. (2018). *Teen tracking app leaks 'thousands' of user passwords.* https://theweek.com/93739/teen-tracking-app-leaks-thousands-of-user-passwords

Watson, M. (2025, November 25). *Young Australians at greatest risk as holiday cyber scams surge. SecurityBrief Australia.* https://securitybrief.com.au/story/young-australians-at-greatest-risk-as-holiday-cyber-scams-surge

3 Protecting your privacy to prevent and mitigate cybersecurity attacks

Lachlan has always dreamed of being the first in his family to go to university. To support his living expenses when he starts his university course next year, the 17-year-old worked part-time at Coles supermarket. His job did not pay much, but seeing his account balance increase over time made him feel confident that, by the time he finished school, he would have enough in his nest egg to support himself while studying to become a cybersecurity professional. He had saved up more than $17,000. Of course, putting aside almost 80% of every dollar he earned in his savings meant he could not buy brand new shoes or order his favourite food, or go out with his friends, but his goal is worth the sacrifice. One day after returning home exhausted from a busy shift, he received an SMS message from his bank that his account had been hacked, and that he needed to log in to block a $10,000 bank transfer. Overwhelmed and consumed with fear, Lachlan clicked on the link in the SMS from his bank, and upon entering his account login details, was prompted to enter the verification code that the bank texted him. As his heart raced and panic took hold, he entered the verification code. Within a split second of entering the six-digit code, he received another SMS message confirming that his $5,000 transfer to a CBA bank account had been successful. 'This can't be right' he thought to himself. Confused and distressed, he logged on to his account by entering the bank's URL. To his shock, he discovered that his account balance was missing $5,000. It was at that moment that he realised he had been scammed. The experience was so humiliating that Lachlan decided not to tell his parents or friends about it. Sadly, when he went to his bank branch and explained the situation and showed them the SMS messages, the bank refused to compensate him for the stolen money because, as far as the bank was concerned, it was a legitimate transaction. Lachlan was devastated that his stolen money could not be recovered. The loss, the shame, and the how it happened questions made him lose sleep. How did the cyber criminal manage to send him an SMS using his genuine bank phone number? How did the

DOI: 10.4324/9781003681731-4

cyber criminal manage to make their SMS messages appear in the same conversation as the previous SMS messages he received from his bank? Where did the cyber criminal get his mobile number from? How did the cyber criminal know he had an account with his bank?

Teens and online experiences with cybersecurity threats

Recent research shows that teenagers are experiencing cybersecurity threats far more often than many realise. Social media platforms are now one of the most common entry points for scams, with around one in four teens aged 13–17 reporting that they have been targeted or scammed online, often through fake online stores, giveaways, or messages that appear to come from other teens. These scams don't always look suspicious at first, as many are designed to feel friendly, familiar, or low risk, which makes them easy to fall for, especially when money, popularity, or urgency is involved.

Teenagers today navigate a digital landscape filled with significant privacy risks, including many they are unaware of. A key concern is photo and video metadata. A 2022 study found that 60% of teens do not realise that the photos and videos they share contain embedded metadata, such as location, timestamps, and device details, that can expose personal information and increase the risk of identity theft. Teens who post images online are highly likely to share at least one photo with geotags or other identifiable details, inadvertently revealing their location. Even seemingly harmless posts, such as a "first day of school" picture or a work pass from a part-time job, can unintentionally compromise personal privacy and safety.

Social media further amplifies these risks. A 2023 study found that 74% of teens have public profiles, making their personal data easily accessible to advertisers, cyber criminals, and predators. In 2024, research revealed that 39% of teens had shared personal identifiers, such as full names, school locations, or dates of birth, without fully understanding the privacy implications. In Australia, up to 60% of teenagers aged 14–17 have public profiles, and one in three admit to sharing personal details openly, significantly increasing their vulnerability to security and privacy breaches. In 2022, 1.7 million US children fell victim to data breaches, highlighting the real-world consequences of inadequate privacy protections.

They take advantage of teens not having but wanting money

Another growing concern is identity misuse and fraud. Young people are increasingly targeted because their personal information is valuable and often goes unnoticed when misused. Research shows that teens may not realise they have been affected until years later, when fraudulent accounts or debts appear in their name. This risk is amplified by the amount of personal data teens share online, often unknowingly, through photos, bios, gaming accounts, and everyday app use.

Rochelle's story is one we could all fall victim to. When she was just 15 years old, she was approached on Instagram by someone offering an easy way to make money by becoming a "money mule", essentially letting criminals use her bank account to move illicit funds. At the time, she had no money, so the promise of a few hundred pounds in exchange for sharing her bank details seemed tempting. However, it was a scam aimed at her. The criminals laundered money through her account, withdrew the funds, and Rochelle received nothing. Her bank later questioned the unusual activity and blocked her account. She described feeling humiliated and embarrassed, believing she had been tricked, and noted that many of her friends, including a sibling, had experienced similar scams.

Financial losses usually cannot be recovered

Recovering funds lost to online scams remains a significant challenge, especially for teenagers. An estimated 87% of victims do not report incidents, often due to embarrassment or a lack of awareness about reporting mechanisms, making it difficult to fully assess financial losses among young people. Moreover, across all age groups, recovery rates remain exceptionally low, with only 7% of victims successfully reclaiming lost funds. This highlights the severity of financial risks tied to online privacy breaches and underscores the need for stronger digital literacy programmes and proactive security measures to better protect teenagers in the digital world.

An Australian teenager lost $37,000 in a matter of seconds after falling victim to a sophisticated phone scam. The teen received a call from someone impersonating a bank representative who claimed suspicious activity had been detected on their account. Using urgency, fear, and official-sounding language, the scammer convinced the teen to quickly approve transactions and share security details, which the teen did, believing they were protecting their money. By the time the call ended, the funds had already been transferred and were unrecoverable. The case highlights how even confident, digitally capable teens can be overwhelmed by high-pressure scams that exploit trust, authority, and panic, demonstrating how fast financial damage can occur once a scammer gains psychological control.

Social media is where you are most targeted

Beyond privacy concerns, teenagers face increasing cyber threats, including phishing scams, identity theft, and social engineering attacks. Research shows that 25% of 13- to 17-year-olds have experienced online scams or fraud. Contrary to common perceptions, identity theft among children is often committed by someone they know, as 75% of children's identity fraud cases involve a relative or a family acquaintance. Additionally, inexperience can make teens an easy target. Two-thirds of individuals aged 15 and over have been exposed to scams, with those under 25 losing over $210 million in 2022 alone. Young people remain a prime target, with scammers adapting to newer platforms like Snapchat and TikTok. However, Facebook and Instagram continue to be the most common platforms where teens report financial losses, particularly from fake online stores or fraudulent ticket sales.

Teens are failing to protect themselves

Despite growing concerns, many teenagers fail to take meaningful protective action. While a large percentage worry about how social media platforms collect and use their data, only 21% understand the privacy policies they agree to, and just 26% actively adjust their privacy settings. This gap between awareness and action, known as the "privacy paradox", suggests that while young users recognise the risks of oversharing, they struggle to implement effective safeguards. The complexity of privacy settings, misleading platform policies, and the convenience of sharing personal information all contribute to this inaction.

Read more information on the privacy paradox and inadvertently sharing sensitive information online in Chapter 2: Smartphone Settings and Your Identifying Information

Despite these risks, many teens feel confident in their ability to spot scams, believing that being "tech-savvy" offers protection. However, studies consistently show a gap between confidence and reality. Scammers are adapting quickly, using AI, newer platforms, realistic profiles, and emotional manipulation to exploit trust. Together, these trends show that online threats are not rare or unlikely events for teenagers, as they are a common part of today's digital world, making awareness, critical thinking, and early action essential skills for staying safe online.

Social engineering and online cyber threats

So, what made Lachlan vulnerable to the scam? It started when he shared a photo of his work pass on social media after getting a job at Coles. Unbeknownst to him, scammers had been tracking his online activity ever since.

Later, he received a friend request from someone claiming they had lost their phone and created new accounts. They messaged him, casually asking details about his part-time job. They even inquired about his bank, pretending they were looking for similar work. What Lachlan didn't realise was that he had been targeted through social engineering tactics for quite some time.

Social engineering is a form of manipulation or deception that tricks you into divulging confidential information, performing actions, or making decisions that may compromise your security. It often exploits human psychology and trust rather than relying on technical hacking methods. Social engineers use tactics such as impersonating trusted individuals or organisations, creating a sense of urgency, or appealing to emotions to manipulate you into revealing sensitive information, such as passwords, financial details, or access to systems.

Common examples of social engineering include pretexting and the Theory of Influence, where an attacker creates a false sense of legitimacy, where they use baiting promises to lure you into compromising your data.

Scam and cyber threat victims are often trusting, follow processes well, enjoy interacting online, and think it won't happen to them. Predators manipulate these factors to create urgency, trust, and compliance. Scammers exploit human psychology, not just technology. Victims aren't "stupid"; they are being manipulated by trained attackers using psychological triggers that anyone can fall for.

Pretexting attacks

The use of an excuse or a story to launch social engineering attacks is called pretexting. Pretexting is a social engineering technique where attackers fabricate a scenario or impersonate a trusted figure to manipulate you into revealing sensitive information, such as passwords, financial details, or personal data. This is essentially the script the attackers will be following.

Scammers often pose as bank officials, employers, or friends, using well-crafted lies to gain trust and exploit their targets. They research their

What is the playbook of a pretexting attack?

1 **Research & Reconnaissance:** The scammer starts by quietly gathering information about you. This might come from your social media posts, photos, comments, bios, or even data from past breaches. Details like your school, workplace, hobbies, friends, or the bank you use help them build a story that feels personal and believable.

2 **Building Trust:** Next, they pretend to be someone you're likely to trust, such as your bank, a delivery company, your employer, a teacher, or even a friend who says they've "lost their phone". Because the message sounds familiar and uses details about your life, it lowers your guard and makes the interaction feel safe.

3 **Creating Urgency:** To stop you from thinking things through, the scammer creates pressure. They might say your account has been compromised, a payment is pending, or something bad will happen if you don't act immediately. Urgency triggers panic and fear, making it harder to spot red flags or ask for help.

4 **Extracting Information:** Once you're worried and trusting them, the scammer asks for sensitive information, such as one-time passcodes, passwords, banking details, or approval of a transaction. Because the request feels official and urgent, many people comply without realising they're being manipulated.

5 **Exploiting the Data:** After they get what they want, the scammer uses the information to steal money, take over accounts, commit identity theft, or target you again. In some cases, they may sell your details to other criminals, leading to ongoing scams long after the original incident.

Check-in: Are you at risk of experiencing pretexting?

❒ **They already seem to know personal details about you**
They mention your job, school, bank, recent posts, or friends, even though you never gave them that information.

❒ **They contact you unexpectedly**
The message, call, or DM comes out of nowhere, and you weren't expecting to hear from them.

❒ **They claim to be someone "official"**
They say they're from your bank, a delivery company, tech support, your employer, or a platform like Instagram or Snapchat.

❒ **They create urgency or pressure**
They say things like "Act now", "Your account will be locked", "This must be fixed immediately", or "Don't tell anyone".

❒ **They ask for sensitive information**
They request passwords, one-time codes, banking details, approval of a transaction, or copies of ID, even if it sounds routine.

❒ **They move the conversation quickly**
They push you to switch from email to text, from social media to WhatsApp, or from chat to a phone call.

❒ **They try to make you feel scared, embarrassed, or responsible**
They use fear ("fraud detected"), guilt ("you caused this"), or shame ("this will be exposed") to control your decisions.

❒ **They discourage checking or getting help**
They tell you not to contact your bank directly, not to talk to your parents, or not to hang up.

If you notice even **<u>ONE</u>** of these:
Pause. Don't respond. Don't click links. Don't share anything.
Verify the message through an official app, website, or trusted adult.

victims, often using social media or data breaches to create a convincing story that justifies their request for personal information.

Theory of Influence

The Theory of Influence plays a crucial role in cyber threats and scams, as scammers exploit psychological principles to get you to reveal sensitive information or take harmful actions. Teens can be at higher risk because they are still developing decision-making skills, desire social validation, and have high online engagement. Here is how the Theory of Influence works:

- **Reciprocity** is exploited in giveaway scams, where you feel obligated to provide personal details in exchange for a fake reward.
- **Commitment** and consistency keep you engaged in the scam. By following through, the attackers make you less likely to question fraudulent interactions.
- **Social proof** is used in phishing scams, where fake messages appear to come from trusted sources, making you more likely to comply.
- **Authority** is leveraged in impersonation scams, where attackers pose as banks or government agencies to coerce you to complete urgent actions.
- **Liking** plays a role in romance scams, where you build trust and send money to fraudsters posing as romantic partners.
- **Scarcity** tactics, such as "limited-time offers", pressure you into making impulsive decisions.

For example, here are the sorts of warning signs that someone is using the Theory of Influence on you:

- ☑ **Scarcity:** "Only two spots left, act now to claim your free giveaway!"
- ☑ **Authority:** "I'm from your bank's fraud team, and you need to verify your account immediately".
- ☑ **Social Proof:** "Hundreds of teens have already made money through this, don't be the one who misses out!"
- ☑ **Liking:** "Hey, I love your content! Let's collab on a paid partnership".
- ☑ **Reciprocity:** "You have qualified for a gift, just fill out this quick form to claim it".
- ☑ **Commitment:** "You already shared your email, just one more step to verify your identity".
- ☑ **Trust Manipulation:** "It's me, your friend! I lost my phone, so I'm messaging from a new account".

Example script a scammer may use:

A scammer might call and say, "Hello, this is *[Fake Name]* from *[Your Bank Account]* Fraud Prevention Team. We've detected suspicious activity on your account. A $1,249 charge was attempted at *[Fake Retailer]* just moments ago that seems suspicious compared to your normal transactions based on your history. To ensure your account remains secure, we need you to verify whether you authorised this transaction".

(Scammer will pause for victim's response, and if they deny the charge, the scammer continues to build urgency.)

Scammer: "Since you did not authorise this, we need to act quickly. To prevent further unauthorised transactions, I'll send you a security verification code via SMS. Please read it back to me so we can secure your account immediately".

(The scammer actually triggers a legitimate two-factor authentication (2FA) code request from the real bank, then tricks the victim into reading it aloud and giving them access to the account.)

How are cyber-attacks executed?

From a technical perspective, the scam for which Lachlan fell victim involved several cyber-attacks, including social engineering, spoofing, phishing, website mirroring, man-in-the-middle attacks, and identity theft. Advances in AI have made these types of cyber-attacks faster, more convincing, and easier than ever for scammers to launch at scale.

Spoofing makes it easy to pretend to be someone legitimate

Lachlan is active on social media, especially Facebook. He shares updates about his life regularly on the platform. His Facebook profile is public, which means his status updates are not only seen by his friends but by anyone who looks him up. His latest Facebook activity was a post in which he shared with his friends his disappointment with his bank. With his mobile number appearing in the Contact Info under the About section of his profile, it was easy for the attacker to send him an SMS message through his bank. This attack is called SMS spoofing.

Spoofing is deceiving by impersonating someone else's identity. Spoofing can happen through all types of contact points, such as SMS, email, and even phone numbers that appear to be from a real company. In this case, the scammer "spoofed" the SMS message header from his bank and sent the victim fake messages about his bank account "being hacked" in the same message thread as the genuine messages the victim had received from his bank before. The attacker was able to do that by using a spoofing tool or service to set the "From" number (sender phone number) to any number they chose, in this case, the victim's bank phone number.

Phishing and website mirroring make it easy to steal your data

By including a link in the text message to direct a recipient to a fake website, a mirror of their bank's website, the attacker attempted a phishing attack, or more accurately, a smishing attack, since this phishing was executed using SMS messages. Generally speaking, phishing is a technique used to obtain information through deception using electronic communications. You might encounter phishing attempts through email or instant messaging. You might also encounter it in the social media platforms you use. In addition, it is incredibly easy to create a mirror website of a legitimate commercial entity. Even an unskilled attacker can launch a website mirroring (or website cloning) attack on a legitimate website.

An attacker can use a simple tool such as HTTrack to clone a legitimate website by downloading all its HTML, images, CSS, JavaScript, and other files. HTTrack can be launched from any operating system environment, including a Kali Linux box, which is the most popular box for hacking. In the case of a fake bank website, the attacker needs only a legitimate site's front end and the bank login page. Once the attacker downloads a copy of the legitimate bank pages, they can then edit the bank login form actions to make it collect user credentials in plain text. The attacker can now host these cloned bank pages on their web server. The attacker can use a similar domain name to the legitimate one to trick the victim into thinking the bank website is genuine.

Typosquatting, man-in-the-middle (MITM), and identity theft make it hard to tell it's not legitimate

In this instance, the attacker does not even need to register this domain name, in which case this would have been a form of Typosquatting. The attacker can just use, for example, for anz.com.au, αnz.com.au, where the "a" here is a Greek α.

When the victim clicks the link in the spoofed SMS message and enters their login details in the fake bank login page, the attacker uses these credentials to log in to the victim's legitimate bank website. This attack is called a man-in-the-middle (MITM) attack. In this case, the attacker positions themselves between the victim and their legitimate bank, neither of whom knows they are communicating via the attacker.

The attack can also be considered a form of identity theft. The attacker stole the login credentials of the victim and presented themselves (impersonated) to the victim's actual bank as the victim by entering those stolen credentials.

How to avoid falling victim to cyber-attacks?

Lachlan could not have predicted the sophistication of the cyber scam he fell victim to, but there were early warning signs that, if recognised, might have reduced the risk. Like many teenagers, he trusted the situation because it appeared urgent, official, and familiar. Knowing the signs that scammers use puts you one step ahead of them.

1 Ensure you adopt a zero trust approach and verify EVERYTHING

When it comes to using computing technology, you should adopt a zero trust approach. To avoid falling victim to an SMS spoofing attack, don't trust the Caller ID alone and never ring a business entity using the phone number included in an SMS message they sent you. You should always verify the information through official channels. Always call your bank from the bank app because you are already identified. Never use a number in a text or in an email. Only use the phone number listed on their official website, which you would have visited via their official bank app, by typing the correct domain name in your computer browser, or by searching for the correct validated link.

Before providing any confidential information via a website, such as login details, you should always check that the connection is secure, over https as denoted by the yellow lock, and that a valid certificate has been issued to the site or business entity you are visiting. This not only ensures that the website is legitimate, but also that any confidential information you provide via your browser will be encrypted as it travels to the website server.

2 Use trusted apps from verified providers

Generally speaking, accessing your bank account via your smartphone's official bank app is considered more secure than visiting your bank website via your computer browser. This is because your smartphone is less likely to be infected with malware compared to your computer. More importantly, banks invest a huge amount of money to ensure their apps are secure, and so as long as you download the correct bank app from a trusted source, then the risk of a phishing attack is reduced every time you go outside the borders of your official bank app to your bank website.

> **Important note about links**: Banks never include contact details in texts anymore to assist you in avoiding falling victim to scams. Banks also advise their customers to call only the number on their bank card or the number on their official website.

3 Never click on links in SMS or emails

To avoid falling victim to a phishing attack, you should never click on any links you receive in an SMS message (or in most cases, in an email message), especially if this message is unsolicited. Clicking on such links can direct you to a fake website or a phishing site, or worse, can infect your computer or device with malicious malware or ransomware. Instead of clicking links in SMS messages, you should verify the information through official channels.

4 Always enable multi-factor authentication (MFA)

You should always enable two-factor authentication using known authentication apps, such as those from Google or Microsoft. These are generally preferred over SMS authentication because the codes are generated locally, making them harder to intercept than unencrypted codes sent via SMS messages. Two-factor authentication gives you another layer of protection when identifying yourself to websites of commercial entities. In addition to claiming who you are (your username) and proving who you are (your password), the commercial entity is assured it is you because of the thing you have (your smartphone). Implementing these measures provides broader protection and can significantly reduce the risk of other cyber-attacks, including website mirroring and man-in-the-middle techniques.

5 Never share your personal details online

Identity theft is on the rise. The 249,448 scams reported in 2024 resulted in losses worth $318,762,688. In addition, 18,512 of these scams involved identity theft. The total loss to these identity theft scams was $8,098,468. There are many benefits of actively participating in social media. Regularly posting social media status updates has been found to benefit a user's well-being. However, leaving your social media profiles public can make you vulnerable to identity theft scams.

As Lachlan's story shows, the attacker needed only Lachlan's mobile number, which Lachlan publicly listed in the Contact Info under the About section of his Facebook profile, and which bank held his money. For this reason, it is not advisable to leave your social media accounts publicly accessible. The latest cyber-attacks on large companies, such as mobile phone, health insurance, and healthcare groups, mean your sensitive personal information is most likely already floating on the dark web. Making your social media profiles open just gives attackers another source of information about you, which they can leverage to tailor the pretext to attack you.

What to do if you have fallen victim to a cyber scam?

Lachlan could not tell his parents, caregiver, or friends about falling victim to a cyber scam because he was ashamed of himself. But he should not have felt ashamed. There is no shame in falling victim to a scam. It can happen to anyone, as evidenced by the more than 1.3 million Australians who have reported getting scammed.

1 Assess the impact and ongoing risks

The first and most important step is to calmly assess and review where your identity or account information may still be at risk. Immediate actions that must be undertaken as soon as possible are:

- **Stop communication** – Cease all contact with the scammer to prevent further manipulation. Block all contact from the scammer and do not send any more money to them under any circumstances.

- **Change passwords** – Immediately update passwords for compromised accounts, using strong, unique passwords for each site.
- **Enable multi-factor authentication (MFA)** – Activate MFA on all accounts to add an extra layer of security.
- **Continue to check bank accounts** – Monitor transactions for any unauthorised activity and contact the bank immediately to report fraud using the numbers on their official website or from the bank app, because you are already identified.
- **Remove any personal information online** – Ensure removal of any contact information on all social media or other online profiles.
- **Report the scam or identity theft to:**
    - All banks or payment providers that were used as part of the scam or could be at risk of someone using your identity.
    - The relevant cyber crime authority in your country. Search online for your government's official website.
    - The police or local cyber crime unit.
    - The social media platform or any apps where the scam occurred. Report any profiles used to contact you.
    - Scam reporting agencies like ScamWatch (Australia), Action Fraud (United Kingdom), or the FBI's IC3 (United States).

2 If you've paid a scammer

If you've sent money to a scammer, act quickly by following these steps:

- **Credit or Debit Card** – Get in touch with your bank or card provider immediately to report the scam and try to reverse the payment.
- **Money Transfer** – Reach out to the wire transfer service or your bank to see if the transaction can be stopped.
- **Money Transfer App** – Report the scam directly to the app provider.
- **Unauthorised Transfer** – If money was taken from your account without permission, report it to your bank immediately and ask for any further transactions to be stopped.
- **Cryptocurrency** – Notify the platform or exchange you used to send the funds.
- **Cash** – If it was sent through the mail or a courier service, contact Australia Post or the delivery provider to check if it can be intercepted.
- **Gift Card** – Contact the company that issued the card to report the fraud.

> **Acting quickly is essential**: The sooner you report fraud or identity theft, the greater your chances of minimising further damage.

3 If someone has gained access to your computer or phone

Cyber threats can include impersonation of internet or phone service providers, claiming there's a technical issue that requires remote access to your device. Once inside, they may install malware to steal passwords, financial details, or other sensitive data.

What to do if your computer or phone has been accessed:

- Immediately disconnect from the internet to prevent further access.
- Update and run a full scan using reputable security software to detect malware or suspicious activity.
- Contact your phone or internet provider to report the incident and check for unauthorised changes.
- For added security, consider having an IT professional inspect your devices to ensure they are free from malware and vulnerabilities.

If you need further assistance, most government agencies worldwide offer cybersecurity hotlines that provide expert advice, support, and guidance. Do not hesitate to reach out if you need help, as understandably, this can be extremely traumatic and confronting. There are many good online support options available to you. Always tell someone if you are scared, stressed, worried, or concerned about what has happened. For example, the following sites have excellent resources for support:

- Australia: Beyond Blue at https://www.beyondblue.org.au
- United Kingdom: Childline at https://www.childline.org.uk
- United States: Cybersmile at https://www.cybersmile.org

Search online for: "[Your country] reporting online scams"; "[Your country] online cyber help"; "What to do if experienced cyber threat"

Conclusion

This chapter focused on protecting privacy and security to prevent cybersecurity attacks. Cybersecurity attacks are a real threat and can happen to you. It is important that you protect your privacy on social media. Do not leave your social media accounts public. It is also important that you don't post sensitive information that can be used to target you, such as your full name, complete date of birth, residential address, mobile number, or information about your health or financial transactions. More importantly, spend some time going through your social media privacy settings. Check things like who can see your future posts, who can see your friend's list, who can look you up using your email or phone number, and who can tag you. There are several steps that you can take to prevent attackers from targeting you: (1) Do not click on any links in SMS messages (or open any attachments) or call a phone number listed in an SMS message. (2) Enable two-factor authentication (2FA) for all social media platforms and websites of commercial entities, especially your banks. (3) Watch for the common signs of a scam in the messages you receive (social media, SMS, email). This chapter also outlines steps on what to do if you have fallen victim to a cybersecurity scam.

Key terms

- SMS = short message service
- Typosquatting
- Sextortion
- Money mule
- Social engineering
- Privacy paradox
- Pretexting
- Theory of Influence
- Cyber-attacks
- Scammer
- Spoofing
- Phishing
- Website mirroring/cloning
- Man-in-the-middle (MITM)
- Zero trust approach
- Multi-factor authentication (MFA)

Bibliography

Allstate Identity Protection. (2025, August 28). *Steps to help shield teens from identity theft.* https://www.allstateidentityprotection.com/content-hub/steps-to-help-shield-teens-from-identity-theft

Australian Competition and Consumer Commission. (2020). *Gen Z: The fastest growing victims of scams.* https://www.accc.gov.au/media-release/gen-z-the-fastest-growing-victims-of-scams

Australian Competition and Consumer Commission. (2023). *Targeting scams: Report of the ACCC on scams activity 2022.* https://www.accc.gov.au/system/files/Targeting%2Bscams%2B2022.pdf

Australian Competition and Consumer Commission. (2026). *Targeting scams report 2025.* https://www.accc.gov.au/about-us/publications/serial-publications/targeting-scams-reports-on-scams-activity/targeting-scams-report-of-the-national-anti-scam-centre-on-scams-data-and-activity-2025

Calvin, A., Lenhart, A., Hasse, A., Mann, S., & Robb, M.B. (2025). *Teens, trust, and technology in the age of AI: Navigating trust in online conten*

Federal Bureau of Investigation. (n.d.). *Financially motivated sextortion crimes targeting minors.* https://www.fbi.gov/how-we-can-help-you/scams-and-safety/common-frauds-and-scams/sextortion/financially-motivated-sextortion

Federal Trade Commission. (2024). *A look behind the screens.* https://www.ftc.gov/system/files/ftc_gov/pdf/Social-Media-6b-Report-9-11-2024.pdf

Forrit Credit Union. (2023, December 8). *Gen Z and scams.* https://www.forritcu.org/gen-z-and-scams/

Goldberg, T. (Kitten). (2022, October 26). *Child identity fraud: The perils of too many screens and social media* [White paper]. https://javelinstrategy.com/whitepapers/child-identity-fraud-perils-too-many-screens-and-social-media

Javelin Strategy & Research. (2022). *17 million US children fell victim to data breaches, according to Javelin's 2022 child identity fraud study.* https://javelinstrategy.com/press-release/17-million-us-children-fell-victim-data-breaches-according-javelins-2022-child

Kazlauskas, J. (2023, January 9). *"Nothing left": Teen loses $37,000 falling victim to alleged NAB scam.* News.com.au. https://www.news.com.au/finance/money/nothing-left-teen-loses-37000-falling-victim-to-alleged-nab-scam/news-story/401d4fe9d8a00fdab2cd8e19fa65bfac

Kelly, G., Graham, J., & Garton, S. (2023). *2023 State of Kids' privacy: Who is monetizing our data? A general lack of transparency leads to a confusing landscape*, San Francisco, CA: Common Sense Media.

Mozilla Foundation. (2023, February 23). *Mozilla study: Data privacy labels for most top apps in Google Play Store are false or misleading.* https://foundation.mozilla.org/en/privacynotincluded/articles/mozilla-study-data-privacy-labels-for-most-top-apps-in-google-play-store-are-false-or-misleading/

Murphy, H. (2024, August 20). *ASIC report finds most bank scam victims bear the burden.* ABC News. https://www.abc.net.au/news/2024-08-20/asic-report-finds-most-bank-scam-victims-bear-the-burden/104247426

National Australia Bank. (n.d.). *How to keep your money and accounts safe.* https://www.nab.com.au/about-us/security/account-security-tips

Ofcom. (2023). *Online Nation 2023 report.* https://www.ofcom.org.uk/siteassets/resources/documents/research-and-data/online-research/online-nation/2023/online-nation-2023-report.pdf

Ofcom. (2026). *Children and parents: Media use and attitudes report 2026.* https://www.ofcom.org.uk/siteassets/resources/documents/research-and-data/media-literacy-research/children/2026-children-and-parents-report/children-and-parents-media-use-and-attitudes-report-2025 6.pdf?v=418231

Ofcom. (2026, May 26). *Children and parents: Media use and attitudes report 2024.* https://www.ofcom.org.uk/media-use-and-attitudes/media-habits-children/childrens-media-lives

Office of the Australian Information Commissioner. (2023). *Australian community attitudes to privacy survey 2023*, Office of the Australian Information Commissioner, Australian Government.

Office of the Australian Information Commissioner. (n.d.). *What is personal information?* https://www.oaic.gov.au/privacy/your-privacy-rights/your-personal-information/what-is-personal-information

Pew Research Center. (2012, July 11). *Teens 2012: Truth, trends, and myths about teen online behavior.* https://www.pewresearch.org/internet/2012/07/11/teens-2012-truth-trends-and-myths-about-teen-online-behavior/

Pew Research Center. (2022, August 10). *Teens, social media and technology 2022.* https://www.pewresearch.org/internet/2022/08/10/teens-social-media-and-technology-2022/

Raising Children Network. (2025). *Online safety for teenagers.* https://raisingchildren.net.au/teens/entertainment-technology/cyberbullying-online-safety/internet-safety-teens

Shaw, A. (2024, June 14). *Attempted kidnapper used Snapchat's location sharing to track down victim.* FOX Carolina. https://www.foxcarolina.com/2024/06/13/attempted-kidnapper-used-snapchats-location-sharing-track-down-victim

Washo, A. H. (2021). An interdisciplinary view of social engineering: A call to action for research. *Computers in Human Behavior Reports,* 4, 100126. https://doi.org/10.1016/j.chbr.2021.100126

WeProtect Global Alliance (2025). *Global Threat Assessment 2025, Preventing technology-facilitated child sexual exploitation and abuse: From insights to action.* https://www.weprotect.org/globalthreat-assessment-25/

Westpac Banking Corporation. (2024, September 6). *One in four teens fall victim to social media scams.* https://www.westpac.com.au/about-westpac/media/media-releases/2024/6-september/

White, M. (2019, February 8). *Revealed: How fraudsters are scamming teenage money mules on Instagram and Snapchat.* Sky News. https://news.sky.com/story/revealed-how-fraudsters-are-scamming-teenage-money-mules-on-instagram-and-snapchat-11630666

Wolbers, H., Cubitt, T., Napier, S., Cahill, M., Nicholas, M., Burton, M., & Giunta, K. (2025). Sexual extortion of Australian adolescents: Results from a national survey. *Trends & Issues in Crime and Criminal Justice* no. 712, Canberra: Australian Institute of Criminology. https://doi.org/10.52922/ti77819

4 Becoming resilient to cyberbullying and trolling

Warning: This anecdote contains language that some readers may find offensive. If this applies to you, skip this section and go to the next.

"Why do the police want to speak to me about you? What have you done?" Rod asked his son as he placed the phone on the kitchen bench. When he did not receive a response, Rod repeated the question louder. "Nothing, I have not done anything wrong, leave me alone, can't you see I am in the middle of a game with my friends?" Adrian answered his dad while swiftly pushing back the mic stick (to mute it) and moving the left earpiece to the side so he could hear his dad. "It can't be nothing if the police want to speak to me about you. You must have done something wrong. Are you going to tell me or not?" asked Rod with a stern look and an irritated voice. "Dad!" shouted Adrian. "I told you, I have not done anything wrong. Stop bothering me." … "Thank you for coming," said the police officer to Rod as he closed the door behind him to a tiny interview room. "What is going on?" asked Rod. "We are investigating a bullying incident at your son's school, and I am afraid there is evidence that suggests your son may have been involved in it," the police officer replied as he pulled a chair and sat on it. "You brought me to the police station late on a Friday afternoon just to tell me that my son may have been involved in a bullying incident!" Rod responded to the police officer, clearly agitated. "Mate, we take bullying incidents seriously," the police officer interrupted. "The victim is fighting for her life at the hospital, and you think this is not a good enough reason for you to come and see us," the police officer angrily replied. … "Did you tell a girl on Snapchat, 'Why don't you go and kill yourself, you fat pig'," Rod asked Adrian the second he stormed into the house. "What, where did this come from?" Adrian responded as he paused the PlayStation. "This is you, isn't it, you f***ing piece of s**t?" Rod furiously asked with his phone's screen right in front of his son's face. Adrian put both his hands over his head in disbelief. The story continues …

DOI: 10.4324/9781003681731-5

Cyberbullying and trolling are one of the biggest risks to your mental health online

Online interactions can be a good way to build social connections from the comfort of your home. However, with the good that can come from interacting with others online, the bad can also result in direct cyberbullying or disruptive trolling, which can have serious emotional and psychological effects. As many as one in six young people aged 11–15 across 44 countries have experienced cyberbullying. In some countries, over half of teens aged 13–17 report having been bullied online, a dramatic rise from just 19% in 2007. In the United States, 46% of teens reported experiencing some form of online harassment. In Australia, it has been shown that 53% of teenagers say they've faced cyberbullying. Among those, one-third reported feeling worthless, one in five felt helpless, and nearly one in six said their mental health declined afterwards. These experiences aren't just unpleasant. They can cause lasting harm and risk to emotional well-being. Research shows strong links between online harassment and increased levels of anxiety, depression, social withdrawal, poor self-image, and even suicidal thoughts. Some studies indicate that nearly 8% of teens who are cyberbullied experience suicidal thoughts.

What is the difference between free speech and trolling?

The key difference is intent and impact: free speech aims to express an idea, while trolling aims to provoke or harm. If something is said mainly to upset, target, or silence someone else, it crosses the line from free expression into online harassment.

Free speech shares ideas and creates diverse views without harm, while trolling targets people with the intent to bully and create harm.

- **Free speech**: is about sharing ideas, opinions, or beliefs, even unpopular ones, without trying to harm others. It's meant to contribute to discussion, debate, or understanding, and it respects that other people are allowed to disagree.
- **Trolling**: is about provoking, upsetting, or humiliating people on purpose. Trolls often post inflammatory, misleading, or cruel comments not to add to the conversation, but to get a reaction, cause drama, or hurt someone.

In Australia, an investigation uncovered social media "bullying pages" on Instagram and TikTok that circulated vulgar slurs and nonconsensual intimate images of school-aged teens. The posts remained active for years, correlating with at least two student suicides (Charlotte O'Brien, 12, and Atreyu McCann, 13). This exposé reveals how social media platforms can enable systemic harassment while protective policies fail to act swiftly enough.

Cyberbullying and trolling are types of online harassment. This means using phones, computers, or other digital tools to repeatedly hurt, upset, or embarrass someone on purpose. It can be done by one person or a group, and it often happens repeatedly.

What is the difference between cyberbullying and trolling?

- **Cyberbullying:** repeated, targeted harassment or activities like spreading rumours or sending hurtful messages, which is often aimed at a specific person or group of people.
- **Trolling:** intentional, provocative, or hate-filled messages meant to upset someone or cause harm.

The effects of both are severe and can include anxiety, depression, poor self-image, social withdrawal, body dysmorphia, and, in extreme cases, self-harm.

Who is most at risk and why?

Teenagers who are part of already marginalised groups or certain age ranges often face higher risks of cyberbullying. A study found that 54% of older teen girls had experienced one of six forms of cyberbullying, compared to 44% of boys in the same age group and 41% of younger teens. Younger teens, especially 12–13-year-olds, are also vulnerable, with over one-third reporting they have been cyberbullied.

LGBTQ+ teens have high rates of online bullying, with reports showing 42% of LGBTQ+ teens have been cyberbullied, more than double the 15% rate among non-LGBTQ+ teens. Research shows transgender and nonbinary students are particularly at risk. Racial and ethnic minority teens also experience elevated levels of cyberbullying.

Factors such as developmental vulnerability, public and relational social interactions online, and prejudiced bias intersect to increase exposure to harmful behaviours.

Did you know? You are most likely to be cyberbullied and trolled by ***someone you know*** rather than strangers online.

Who engages in cyberbullying and trolling, and why?

Most cyberbullying and trolling targeting teens is carried out by peers, not strangers, usually classmates or individuals within the same age group. Perpetrators are frequently students from the same school, social circle, or online community. These individuals may be motivated by a desire for social power, revenge, boredom, or entertainment.

Adolescent boys, especially those who have been victims of trolling themselves, are more likely to engage in trolling behaviours. They often report enjoying the emotional reaction their posts provoke. Cyberbullying can also be reinforced by group dynamics and status games, where young people mimic the behaviours of popular peers or participate to avoid being targeted themselves. Some teens may have low empathy or a limited understanding of the emotional harm their actions can cause, particularly when interactions happen through screens without real-time feedback. Because of this, some online environments, especially ones where people don't face real-life consequences, are more likely to encourage harmful behaviour towards others.

A 20-year-old man in Germany, part of an online grooming network known as "764", was arrested for a campaign of abuse targeting vulnerable children aged 11–15. The individual allegedly coerced a 13-year-old US boy into livestreaming his own suicide and blackmailed multiple victims by recording the abuse. Authorities in Germany, the United States, Canada, and the United Kingdom have linked the suspect to over 120 offences. This unfortunate case highlights the deeply disturbing behaviour and callousness of what people do to others on the internet.

Recent cyberbullying stories from around the world show how serious and damaging online harassment can be for teens. In one widely discussed case, a Netflix documentary (*Unknown Number*) revealed how a teen was relentlessly targeted by a catfish using fake accounts who turned out to be the teen's own mother, showing how one determined troll, especially if it's from a close tie, can cause long-term emotional harm. In another case, a 13-year-old in the United States was charged after creating fake TikTok content to humiliate a peer, highlighting that teens themselves can face real legal consequences for online cruelty.

Other recent stories include teens speaking publicly about the anxiety, fear, and isolation caused by ongoing online abuse, and a shocking case where a young person discovered their cyberbully was someone they trusted at home. Together, these examples show that cyberbullying is not "just drama online"; it can involve deception, persistence, public humiliation, and serious emotional impact, reminding teens why recognising harmful behaviour and getting help early matters.

Why do people bully and troll others online?

Understanding why Adrian behaved cruelly online can help you better respond, protect yourself, and support others. Some people cyberbully or troll online because the internet can make it feel like the normal rules of face-to-face life don't apply, which seems to be relevant to Adrian's situation as well.

In real life, there could be physical or verbal consequences for the person or for others who see the behaviour. Behind a screen, the bully or troll might feel anonymous, powerful, or untouchable, which can lead them to say or do things they'd never do in person. Sometimes it's about chasing attention, laughs, or a reaction, even if it hurts someone else. Others do it to feel in control, to fit in with a certain group, or to put someone down to make themselves feel better. Understanding these motives doesn't excuse the behaviour, but it can help you spot what's going on and protect yourself from it. Although there's never a good reason to cyberbully or troll, psychology helps explain why some people can indulge in these hurtful behaviours.

Hiding behind a screen and online disinhibition

The online disinhibition effect is where anonymity lowers the barrier to harmful behaviours online and emboldens people to act without worrying about immediate consequences. When people can't be seen or identified, they're more likely to say things they would never say face-to-face. Without the usual consequences of real-life interaction, like seeing someone cry or getting in trouble at school, some people feel it is okay to be mean, rude, or outrageous. They might believe their comments "don't really hurt anyone", even though they do. The screen can act like a mask, making it easier to ignore empathy and act without guilt. The power of anonymity makes people act in strange and mean ways.

Why do people act differently online than face-to-face?

People often act differently online than they do in real life because not being face-to-face with someone creates a sense of distance and invisibility. Behind a screen, individuals feel free from everyday social rules and expectations as they don't have to see the person's reaction, worry about being judged in real time, or face direct consequences of what they do or say. This sense of anonymity and disconnection from face-to-face interactions can reduce empathy and increase boldness, making it easier for some people to say or do things online that they would never consider in person. Without the usual social cues or accountability, harmful behaviours like cyberbullying or trolling can feel less serious.

Trying to feel powerful or in control

Many people who cyberbully try to feel strong, popular, or respected, especially if they feel powerless in other areas of their lives. They may have low self-esteem or be dealing with stress, rejection, or pressure. By putting others down, they temporarily feel more important. This is a form of dominance behaviour, where hurting someone else gives them a false sense of control or a feeling that they are better than others.

Revenge or payback

Sometimes people cyberbully because they feel hurt, embarrassed, or excluded, and they want to get even. Maybe they were bullied before, and now they want someone else to feel the same pain. This cycle of harm is known as reactive aggression. While it can come from a place of anger or sadness, it's still wrong and often makes things worse for everyone.

Boredom and thrill-seeking

Some people troll or bully online simply because they're bored. They want a reaction and especially a dramatic one in return. These people, often called internet trolls or keyboard warriors, may post offensive or outrageous comments just to stir up arguments or upset others. They thrive on attention and emotional responses, even if it's negative. Psychologists call this "negative social reward", feeling pleasure from causing discomfort or putting others down.

What is negative social reward?

Negative social reward is when someone feels satisfaction or enjoyment from upsetting, angering, or provoking others. Trolls often seek this kind of reward by causing emotional reactions, even if those reactions are negative, because it gives them a sense of control or attention.

Peer pressure and popularity games

In group chats, gaming platforms, or social media, bullying sometimes becomes part of a group dynamic. Someone might join in just to fit in or avoid becoming the next target. Others might bully to gain "likes", laughs, or social approval. These behaviours are linked to a psychological component of social comparison and the pressure to maintain a certain image online. This kind of group-based bullying can be especially dangerous because it's harder to stop when others remain silent or join in.

What is social comparison?

Social comparison is when people measure their own worth by comparing themselves to others, especially in terms of popularity, appearance, or success. Online, this can lead to jealousy, insecurity, or pressure to act in a certain way to fit in or seem "better" than others.

Lack of empathy or emotional awareness

Some cyberbullies don't understand and sometimes just don't care how much damage they're doing. Especially because they can't see the other person's face or hear their voice, they feel disconnected from the pain they cause. Over time, this emotional distance can lead to a lack of empathy, which means they stop seeing their target as a real person with real feelings. This disconnect is one of the biggest reasons why bullying online can escalate so quickly.

Copying what they see or experience

Many young people who bully both offline and online repeat what they've seen others do or what they have experienced themselves, whether at home, in school, or even on TV or social media. If someone grows up experiencing or watching aggressive or abusive behaviours, they may come to think it's normal. Some may even be victims themselves. This pattern is called modelling, where people imitate behaviours they observe, especially when they see others getting attention or approval for them. When people become so accustomed to experiencing volatile behaviour, they try to recreate the experience for the comfort it brings, because it feels familiar.

Understanding the underlying causes of why Adrian engaged in cyberbullying and trolling does not justify these actions. However, recognising that Adrian's behaviour most likely stems from insecurity, pain, or confusion can provide insights that can help you understand the cause of being attacked. These behaviours are not a reflection of your worth or anything you have done, but rather indicative of the bully's personal struggles and inability to interact appropriately with others.

Individuals, such as Adrian, who engage in online harassment, are typically coping with their own issues and projecting their difficulties onto others. Therefore, it is essential to refrain from responding. Should you ever feel inclined to react negatively online, remember that you possess the ability to choose more constructive behaviours. True strength lies in maintaining dignity and refusing to let others lower your standards.

Check-in: Are you being cyberbullied or trolled?

- ❒ The messages or comments are meant to hurt, embarrass, or upset me
- ❒ It's happening more than once, or the same person keeps coming back
- ❒ The person won't stop even after I ignore or block them
- ❒ I feel anxious, angry, scared, or embarrassed after going online
- ❒ They are mocking, threatening, spreading rumours, or telling lies
- ❒ They are trying to provoke a reaction or start drama
- ❒ Fake accounts or anonymous profiles are being used

- ❒ Others are being encouraged to join in or pile on
- ❒ My photos, posts, or words are being shared without my permission
- ❒ I'm starting to avoid apps or people because of it

If you checked **one or more**, you are experiencing online harassment.

Act quickly: if someone won't leave you alone or is exposing your personal information, it's serious, and you need to take action straight away.

How does technology increase the risk of cyberbullying and trolling?

While cyberbullying and trolling were Adrian's fault, technology is not neutral in how it contributes to the culture of bullying or trolling online. Each technology we use comes with certain features that can encourage these behaviours. Cyberbullying and trolling are afforded by certain features inherent in the design of the technologies we use. By afford we mean that the technology is not only facilitating cyberbullying and trolling but also encouraging these behaviours by making them easier or attractive to engage with, or both. For this reason, it is essential to understand how the technology you use enables cyberbullying and trolling.

Anonymity and a lack of accountability functions increase negative interactions

Snapchat's ephemeral messaging feature (i.e., messages disappear after 24 hours from opening unless settings are adjusted) can hide accountability for actions because, with the message disappearing, any evidence of wrongdoing vanishes. Likewise, the anonymity inherent in gaming platforms, such as PlayStation, Discord, and Xbox, coupled with the competitive nature of playing a game with peers, can make users feel disinhibited, turning a game of football into a game of verbal abuse tennis. The back-and-forth exchange of insults, which at the time may sound like banter, can have a huge toll on the mental well-being of the players.

Let us look more closely at some of the social media features that contribute to cyberbullying and trolling behaviours. Snapchat's key feature is that messages posted on it, including snaps and group chats, usually disappear 24 hours after opening, unless the settings are updated. This feature is advantageous for maintaining privacy, because if you shared a photo of yourself that you regret, it won't be there forever; it will be gone, and people will forget about it by the time you wake up. But on the other hand, this self-destructing feature means messages can't be traced and, as indicated above, cannot be used as evidence to make someone accountable for their actions.

That messages self-erase after a while can encourage users to be impulsive in sharing upsetting images of others or share humiliating rumours about them.

Knowing the messages will soon vanish can even make users mean or aggressive towards others, especially if they are anonymous too. If they are anonymous, by creating a fake account, then they are difficult to trace, even if the messages do not disappear. One way around this, of course, is to take a screenshot of the message before it disappears. The person sending the message will get a notification that you have taken a screenshot as evidence. Even if they deny they are the original publishers of the message, they can't deny they at least shared it. You should also avoid engaging with contacts you don't know and don't meet face-to-face, which will solve the anonymity issue.

In multiplayer games, anonymity can be a real issue, though. On a gaming platform like PS5, you receive a request from someone you think you know from school to join your game, but as the game progresses, and they hear your voice, determine your gender, age, and race, the anonymity can embolden them to be mean to you. The anonymity, fast-paced, and competitive nature of gaming are often associated with the exchange of threatening, offensive, and attacking messages. For this reason, you should not play with anyone you don't know in real life. If someone says they know you from school, ask a question only a real classmate would know, like "What class do we have together on Mondays?" It is also worth muting your mic at the beginning as you get a feel for the person you are playing with. The effort to use AI to address hate speech during online games is gaining momentum, but it is challenging considering the interaction is synchronous (real-time) and anonymous.

Allowing fake accounts allows harassment to occur

Instagram is designed for sharing photos and short videos. In addition to its effective and appealing photo and short video feed, Instagram also offers private messaging and self-erasing stories. One troubling feature of Instagram is that it allows anyone to create a fake account to post or comment on other users' photos without revealing their identity.

When users comment on a message (made up of a photo, video, and/or text), like it, or share it, the message's visibility increases, which can make it spread rapidly. Instagram's Public Explore feature, which can turn content considered funny or harmless into viral content, can cause the person about whom the message is shared to be harassed (bullied and trolled) by strangers or peers in their Instagram feed, through direct messaging (DM), or on their school grounds.

Meta, which owns Instagram, has introduced several features to mitigate this problem, such as an AI-powered warning system that alerts users when a post contains a hateful message and natural language filters that help stop the spread of such messages. However, because attackers are creative in using misspelled words, cryptic language or memes (slang, sarcasm, or context), or embedding slurs and insults in images, these messages can escape the filters. This is why researchers have turned their attention to Instagram as a platform where teens experience cyberbullying. So, you need to consider whether the risks are worth it if you want to be on this platform.

TikTok's features can also encourage cyberbullying. The duet feature, for example, which can enable a TikTok user to pair their video with an already published video, can cause a well-intended video to be the subject of ridicule when paired with another video that is aimed to make fun of it. The TikTok incredibly personalised "For You" feed is designed for maximising engagement. TikTok understands users' preferences better than the users themselves. The reason harmful content spirals quickly sometimes is because controversial or sensational content drives strong reactions from other TikTok users, which is why the TikTok algorithms push harmful content to the top, as it creates the most responses. The fear then is that young users treat harmful content as normal.

What is even more concerning is that TikTok has a global reach, making your posts visible to an international audience and potentially allowing anyone, from any jurisdiction, to reach you anonymously. This direct contact with anonymous users can make you especially vulnerable to falling victim to cyberbullying and trolling. Accountability in this case is even trickier because they may reside in a country where anything goes. The good news is that while you have no control over what other users say outside your video feed, you can now approve or block comments in your video feed if they offend you.

Cyberbullies and trolls can use advanced technological capabilities to carry out their cyberbullying and trolling attacks. For example, they can use bots to launch their attacks. A cyberbullying attack coordinated by bots by sending thousands of messages to a victim's feed or as direct messages (DMs) can be devastating to victims because the simultaneous arrival of many messages can amplify the impact of the attack, making the victim feel overwhelmed. Attackers can either automate the sending of messages from multiple fake accounts that they have created or obtain them from an attack-as-a-service provider. These bots can also be used by trolls to mass-tag a victim in abusive posts to embarrass and belittle the victim.

AI tools can exacerbate the problem because they can be socially engineered to auto-generate thousands of harassing or threatening messages to a targeted victim, rendering them powerless. AI tools can mine a victim's social media data (to dig up dirt on them, so to speak), making the attack feel more personal and upsetting. Because AI tools have a better understanding of how moderation filters work, if social media platforms use them, AI tools are in a better position than humans to evade them; for example, by deliberately misspelling words or using different spellings.

How to use technical solutions to protect yourself from falling victim to cyberbullying and trolling

There are several measures you can take to fight back against cyberbullying and trolling, including ensuring you select who sees your content and who can contact you.

1 Ensure effective management of privacy settings

   You can set your privacy and account settings on Snapchat so only your friends or people listed in your contacts can send you messages.

Switch your Facebook and Instagram accounts to private mode so that unknown users can't see your posts. Turn off DMs in Instagram to disable message requests from unknown users. On TikTok, restrict who can DM you or comment on your posts. You are also able to reject friend and follow requests from people you do not know, and block and ignore requests to add you, and can quietly (social media platforms won't tell them) remove existing friends or unfriend them and unfollow them. This will stop them from seeing your content. On all social media platforms, you can block users who you don't want to see your profile, contact you, or even tag you.

Read more information on app privacy settings in Chapter 2: Smartphone Privacy, Security Settings and Your Identifying Information

2 Familiarise yourself with the safety features of apps

Most social media and gaming platforms have built-in safety features. Familiarise yourself with such features so the content you encounter is always right for you. For example, Instagram's comment filter can automatically hide insulting or harassing comments, and you can customise the filter by adding words you don't want to see in your feed. Similarly, TikTok has a filter that can remove profane or abusive content from comments posted on your videos. Game apps like Fortnite block profanity for young users. In-app safety features can also be used to handle bullies. Most social media apps let you block, mute, and report someone bothering you. On Instagram, you can block or mute a harasser, and the app won't notify them. On Instagram, you can also restrict a user's comments so that only the users who posted the comments can see them; no one else. Because a bully can still see the comment they posted, they can't tell that it is hidden from others, and only they can see it.

What to do if you are being bullied and trolled online

1 Don't respond or retaliate

Firing back at a bully might feel tempting, but it often just makes things worse, and it gives them exactly what they want (a reaction). Taking a break or walking away gives you space to cool down, so you don't say something you'll regret or get pulled into a back and forth. Standing up to a bully, especially online, more often just makes them more aggressive. It's usually better to stay calm and completely ignore them. Don't give them what they want.

2 Save the evidence

Take screenshots, record dates, and maintain messages as evidence. Keep a record of any cyberbullying or trolling messages or posts. Save or print copies of emails or online conversations. Preserve text messages on your phone. The type of evidence you should save is:

1 **Screenshots** – Take clear captures of messages, posts, comments, or images, including usernames, timestamps, and any context around them.
2 **Chat logs or message history** – Save full conversations from texts, DMs, or group chats, even if only part of it is cyberbullying or trolling.
3 **URLs/links** – Copy and store direct links to posts, profiles, or videos that contain the cyberbullying or trolling content.
4 **Emails** – Save or forward abusive or threatening emails.
5 **Photos or videos** – Keep copies of any images or videos sent to you or posted publicly about you.
6 **Caller information** – If the cyberbullying involves phone calls, note down numbers, call times, and voicemail messages.
7 **Witness statements** – If friends saw the cyberbullying or trolling happen online, ask if they can confirm what they saw in writing or screenshots.
8 **Platform notifications** – Save push notifications or app alerts that show harmful messages before they get deleted.
9 **Any responses you gave** – Keep records of anything you sent back, to show the full context of the interaction.

This information can be important when reporting incidents of bullying or trolling.

3 Report the bully or troll

All platforms have built-in ways to report bullying or inappropriate behaviour. Social media services and apps must address any complaints and should remove cyberbullying material reported to them. If a social media service fails to remove the material within two days of your report, you can make a complaint to your government cyber-safety website.

Search online for "report social media cyberbullying complaints [*your country*]"; "[your country] online bullying support"

4 Block or mute the person

Use the app or platform's tools to stop contact and ensure they have no way of contacting you:

- ☑ Block the person who is displaying the bullying behaviour
- ☑ Unfriend them
- ☑ Block calls and texts from their number
- ☑ Change your privacy settings

5 Tell someone you trust and get emotional support

You are not alone, and adults can assist you even if it seems they cannot. People who are cyberbullied may feel embarrassed or reluctant to report a bully. There's no need to feel that way. You may hesitate because you are not 100%

sure who is doing the bullying, and you don't think it will make a difference. But bullying can get worse, so it is recommended that you speak with a parent, caregiver, teacher, school counsellor, or helpline. Sometimes the police or other authorities can track down bullies even if they are anonymous, so it's always worthwhile to report it.

Bullying can be very harmful. It is acceptable to feel distressed. Consider discussing your feelings with friends, seeking help from a school counsellor, or reaching out to a teen support service, either by phone or online.

Remember

✓ Don't respond to bullies. Getting a reaction out of you will only encourage them.

✓ Cyberbullies and trolls usually torment multiple people. It is important that you report it not only to help yourself but also to help others.

Search online for "teen help line [*your country*]"; "[your country] online teen mental health support"

Conclusion

Online harassment can have serious emotional and psychological effects, whether through targeted bullying or disruptive trolling behaviour. This chapter teaches teenagers how to recognise cyberbullying, respond safely, and seek help to create safe digital environments. It also distinguishes trolling from free speech, offering guidance on promoting positive online interactions. You can protect yourself from cyberbullying and trolling by properly configuring your privacy and account settings in your social media apps. Measures you can take include restricting who sees your content, and who can contact you, and don't forget you also have the ability to hide or filter out or block content in your feed or chat.

Bullying can be very harmful for your mental health and wellbeing. It is acceptable to feel distressed. Always discuss your feelings with friends or family, seek help from a school counsellor, or reach out to a teen support service either via telephone or online.

Key terms

- Cyberbullying
- Trolling

- Harassment
- Online disinhibition effect
- Negative social reward
- Anonymity
- Verbal abuse tennis
- Fake accounts
- Bots
- Viral
- Global reach

Bibliography

Alfree, C. (2025, September 3). *Florida cyberbullying crimes explained.* First Coast News. https://www.firstcoastnews.com/article/news/crime/florida-cyberbullying-crimes-explained-nassau-county-teen-fake-tik-toks-arrested/77-3d03d52a-1fc4-49c5-8a59-62f400849644

AIHW. (2021, June 25). *Negative online experiences of children and teens.* https://www.aihw.gov.au/reports/children-youth/negative-online-experiences

Anti-Defamation League. (2021). *Online hate and harassment: The American experience 2021.* https://www.adl.org/sites/default/files/pdfs/2022-05/Online%20Hate%20and%20Harassment%202021_042821_V17%282%29.pdf

Artemis Hospitals. (2023, October 12). *The impact of trolling on teen mental health.* https://www.artemishospitals.com/blog/the-impact-of-trolling-on-teen-mental-health

Avast. (2024, August 27). *Key Cyberbullying Statistics for 2025.* https://www.avast.com/c-cyberbullying-statistics

Bottaro, A. (2025, November 14). *Cyberbullying effects and what to do.* Verywell Health. https://www.verywellhealth.com/cyberbullying-effects-and-what-to-do-\5220584

BrightPath Behavioral Health. (2025, June25). *Teenage cyberbullying statistics 2026.* https://www.brightpathbh.com/teenage-cyberbullying-statistics/

Centers for Disease Control and Prevention. (n.d.). *Emotional well-being and suicide risk among American Indian and Alaska Native high school students.* https://www.cdc.gov/yrbs/media/pdf/aian/AIAN_MH_FactSheets508.pdf

Chen, D. (2023, April 23). *Young men more likely to internet troll study finds.* ABC News. https://www.abc.net.au/news/2023-04-22/young-men-more-likely-to-internet-troll-study-finds/102246048

Comparitech. (2021, May 21). *LGBTQ cyberbullying: A guide for parents and educators.* https://www.comparitech.com/blog/vpn-privacy/lgbtq-cyberbullying/

Cuncic, A. (2026, February 25). *The psychology of cyberbullying.* Verywell Mind. https://www.verywellmind.com/the-psychology-of-cyberbullying-5086615

Dasio, S. (2025, June 19). *Police say a German man engaged in cybergrooming and pressured a US teen to kill himself.* AP News. https://apnews.com/article/4047eec634bb2cd52c15a2787126b8d3

DataProt Team. (2023, April 10). *Heart-breaking cyberbullying statistics for 2026.* https://blog.dataprot.net/cyberbullying-statistics

Fernández, M (2025, January 31). *Cyberbullying stats, trends, and insights.* Softonic. https://en.softonic.com/articles/cyberbullying-stats-trends-insights

Gjorgievska, L. (2024, February 8). *Cyberbullying statistics in Australia*. Take a Tumble. https://takeatumble.com.au/insights/lifestyle/cyberbullying-statistics/

Grosse, P. (2026, Feb 12). *Cyberbullying statistics*. ZipDo. https://zipdo.co/cyber-bullying-statistics

Key Healthcare. (2023). *Impact of online harassment on teen mental health*. https://keyhealthcare.com/impact-of-online-harassment-on-teen-mental-health/

KFF (Kaiser Family Foundation). (2023). *Recent trends in mental health and substance use concerns among adolescents*. https://www.kff.org/mental-health/issue-brief/recent-trends-in-mental-health-and-substance-use-concerns-among-adolescents/

Khan, O. (2025, October 22). *Teen speaks out on cyberbullying*. Spectrum News 1. https://spectrumnews1.com/oh/columbus/news/2025/10/22/teen-speaks-out-on-cyberbullying

Korchmaros, J. (2013). Out online: The experiences of lesbian, gay, bisexual and transgender youth on the internet. *Academia.edu*. https://www.academia.edu/94246419/Out_Online_The_Experiences_of_Lesbian_Gay_Bisexual_and_Transgender_Youth_on_the_Internet

PACER Center. (2025, February 28). *Bullying statistics*. https://www.pacer.org/bullying/info/stats/

Patchin, J.W., & Hinduja, S. (2024). *Cyberbullying facts*. Cyberbullying Research Center. https://cyberbullying.org/facts

Piccoli, V., Carnaghi, A., Grassi, M., Stragà, M., & Bianchi, M. (2020). Cyberbullying through the lens of social influence: Predicting cyberbullying perpetration from perceived peer-norm, cyberspace regulations and ingroup processes. *Computers in Human Behavior, 102*, 260–273. https://doi.org/10.1016/j.chb.2019.09.001

Poposki, C. (2025, September 3). *Wild culprit behind gross texts to teenager*. News.com.au. https://www.news.com.au/lifestyle/real-life/news-life/wild-culprit-behind-gross-texts-to-michigan-teenager/news-story/bf1d9cb171096940a57c14fe853ab2fe

Sánchez-Hernández, M.D., Herrera, M.C., Villanueva-Moya, L., & Expósito, F. (2023). Cyberbullying on Instagram: How adolescents perceive risk in personal selfies? *Cyberpsychology: Journal of Psychosocial Research on Cyberspace, 17*(5), Article 2. https://doi.org/10.5817/CP2023 5 2

Schaeffer, K. (2023, November 17). *9 facts about bullying in the U.S.* Pew Research Center. https://www.pewresearch.org/short-reads/2023/11/17/9-facts-about-bullying-in-the-us/

Sproul-Mellis, E. (2025, June 2). *Vile slurs targeting Sydney teens exposed*. Daily Telegraph. https://www.dailytelegraph.com.au/new-south-wales-education/deadly-bullying-pages-targeting-nsw-pupils-left-to-flourish-for-years/news-story/2292226e8d7183162ca782ba0101c6d4

The Trevor Project. (2021, October 14). *Bullying and suicide risk among LGBTQ youth*. https://www.thetrevorproject.org/research-briefs/bullying-and-suicide-risk-among-lgbtq-youth/

12South Recovery. (2024, April 8). *Social media trolls on mental health*. https://12southrecovery.com/articles/social-media-trolls-on-mental-health/

Vogels, E.A. (2022, December 15). *Teens and cyberbullying 2022*. Pew Research Center. https://www.pewresearch.org/internet/2022/12/15/teens-and-cyberbullying-2022/

Wang, L., Jiang, S., Zhou, Z., Fei, W., & Wang, W. (2024). Online disinhibition and adolescent cyberbullying: A systematic review. *Children and Youth Services Review, 156*, 107352. https://doi.org/10.1016/j.childyouth.2023.107352
WebWatcher. (2021, January 21). *LGBTQ youth at greater risk for online bullying.* https://www.webwatcher.com/lgbtq-youth-at-greater-risk-for-online-bullying/
World Health Organization Regional Office for Europe. (2024, March 27). *One in six school-aged children experiences cyberbullying, finds new WHO Europe study.* https://www.who.int/europe/news/item/27-03-2024-one-in-six-school-aged-children-experiences-cyberbullying--finds-new-who-europe-study

5 Protecting yourself from cyberstalking and doxing

While the man who stalked Melanie, the 17-year-old student we met in the chapter on smartphone settings and your identifying information, disappeared after Melanie's mum confronted him in the shopping mall, Melanie's nightmare did not end there. When Melanie blocked the same stalker who pretended to be her Snapchat friend, her Snapchat stalker did the unthinkable. The Snapchat stalker retaliated by creating a website about her in which he detailed not only her full name, home address, school, the park where she takes her dog for a walk and the mall where she goes for shopping, but he also posted photos of her with her friends, which she shared with her best friends, including him before she realised he was an imposter, in strict confidence and in the knowledge that the photos would disappear within 24 hours. In one photo, Melanie could be seen vaping with two of her friends outside the school cafeteria. She found out she had been doxed when the school office called her mum to inform her that her daughter had been suspended for three days for vaping on school grounds. It turned out that one student stumbled upon the site that showed these school students vaping. Concerned about her physical safety, Melanie asked ChatGPT 5 how she could get her personal details and the incriminating photo removed from that website. On this occasion, ChatGPT's response was helpful. The AI agent advised Melanie to report the doxing incident to the eSafety Commissioner, which Melanie did using their website reporting mechanism. Not long after lodging her complaint, Melanie received an update from eSafety, letting her know that they had issued a legal takedown notice to the web hosting service hosting the website. The update asked her to check the offending website in a few days to see if the content had been removed. When Melanie checked the website a few days later, she found that it was no longer reachable. The ISP provider had complied with the legal takedown notice by removing the offending website. Melanie was happy that both the stalking and doxing ordeals appeared to be over.

DOI: 10.4324/9781003681731-6

The rise of cyberstalking and doxing

Cyberstalking and doxing are serious issues that many teens face today. These forms of digital harassment can lead to fear, anxiety, and long-lasting emotional distress. Cyberstalking involves using digital tools to harass, monitor, and control someone, making them feel unsafe. It includes unwanted contact, abusive messages, location tracking, hacking accounts, and interfering with technology. Cyberstalking often aims to scare, shame, or control victims, and can escalate to physical threats. It commonly occurs in domestic violence situations, and cutting off digital access doesn't stop the abuse. Teens who experience cyberstalking can become disengaged from school and education.

Doxing (or doxxing) refers to the practice of gathering and disseminating an individual's personal information with the intention of shaming, embarrassing, exposing, or intimidating them. This information may be sourced from private records but is frequently obtained from public sources. The term originates from the phrase "dropping dox (documents)" and describes a tactic that has developed into a form of online harassment, which may escalate into stalking or other criminal activities.

What is the difference between cyberstalking and doxing?

- **Cyberstalking**: Cyberstalking is when a person keeps constant track of you online in a way that makes you feel uncomfortable, worried, or threatened.
- **Doxing**: Doxing (or doxxing) is the action or process of collecting and disseminating someone's personal information to shame, embarrass, expose, or intimidate them.

In the United States, a scary case showed just how serious cyberstalking can get. A 45-year-old man, Timothy Nielsen, became obsessed with a young girl after watching her arts and crafts videos on YouTube when she was just six. He started leaving creepy comments, and even after her channel was taken down, he followed her across other social media platforms using fake accounts. Years later, when she was 12, he travelled from Oregon to Ohio and went door to door in her neighbourhood trying to find her. Luckily, the police caught him before he could get to her, and he was sentenced to four-and-a-half years in prison. This real-life case is a chilling reminder that some online stalkers will stop at nothing to harass someone and that online harassment can lead to serious real-world danger.

Who is most at risk of cyberstalking and doxing?

It appears that children and young people are more likely to experience cyberstalking than adults and older people. A review of cyberbullying incidents in the last five years shows an average victimisation rate of 33% among adolescents and children. Studies show that a substantial number of teens have been cyberstalked, with some studies reporting rates as high as 62% among adolescents aged 12–16. Globally, approximately 7.5 million people experience cyberstalking each year, with 80% of victims tracked using technology.

Recent research shows that online harassment and stalking behaviours are very common among young people. Surveys of teens aged 13–17 in the United States found that nearly half (46%) have experienced some form of online harassment, including repeated unwanted messages or rumours that can be part of stalking behaviour, and about 7% reported having explicit images shared without their consent, a form of doxing and sexual violation. Other studies show that many teenagers have seen or been directly targeted by online harassment and cyberstalking, with almost 48% of teens reporting they have witnessed stalking or harassment behaviours online, and about 26% saying they've been called offensive names repeatedly, which often overlaps with cyberstalking situations.

Cyberstalking and doxing happen where teens spend most of their time online

Many teens experience cyberstalking and doxing through the very places they spend the most time online, especially on social media platforms. Research shows that a large share of online harassment happens where teens interact with friends and followers, post photos, or share parts of their lives. Teens who are online constantly, especially on platforms like Instagram, Snapchat, TikTok, and Facebook, are more likely to face multiple forms of online abuse because those spaces make personal details easier to access and misuse.

Online gaming communities are another common environment where teens experience harassment that can lead to stalking or doxing. Studies of cyberstalking data show that while social media is the main place for this harm, gaming platforms and group chats are also hotspots for hurtful behaviour, including offensive messages, targeted harassment, and attempts to share or pressure for personal information. A global sample found that teens encounter harassment not just in comments and direct messages but also while playing online games, and nearly one in five teens report being called offensive names in those spaces.

In 2024, a 15-year-old gamer got into an argument with someone in a multiplayer lobby, and then everything spiralled out of control. The other players somehow found his IP, then his real name and home address, and posted it publicly online. For weeks afterwards, strangers flooded his house with dozens of unsolicited food deliveries every day, sometimes up to 50 orders a day, leaving his front yard and porch buried in packages and forcing him and his family to answer the door multiple times a day to stop the chaos. Even after it faded, the boy said he remained in a constant state of alert, worried that those same strangers still knew exactly where he lived and could return.

Cyberstalking is gendered

One in four females and one in five males have experienced cyberstalking before the age of 17. Research indicates that cyberstalking is gendered, which is consistent with patterns of family violence, sexual violence, and harassment. It is often carried out by men against women and girls. Around 70% of the online harm reports that eSafety receives are from Australian women and girls. While technology can empower women and girls, in this instance, technology has exacerbated harmful, sexist, misogynistic, and violent online behaviour. Men also experience cyberstalking. Some research suggests that women cyberstalk more than men, and that men report more online victimisation than women.

Women and girls are often targeted more frequently and more intensely than males, with surveys finding that women are far more likely than men to experience technology-facilitated abuse, including threats, intimidation, and online harassment. In one large study, women were about twice as likely as men to fear for their safety after online abuse, and many reported being targeted by someone else's technology rather than in person. Young people, especially those aged 16–24, also face higher rates of cyberstalking than older age groups, and gender minorities and lesbian, gay and bisexual teens can be even more affected than their heterosexual peers. These patterns make it clear that cyberstalking is not just a "digital inconvenience", it's a real and gendered form of online harm that can affect people differently based on age, gender, and identity.

> **Did you know?** Cyberstalking is frequently associated with incidents of offline stalking, which can pose significant threats to your personal safety.

Who is doing cyberstalking and doxing?

Cyberstalkers can be peers, ex-partners, or anonymous individuals who exploit online platforms to harass and intimidate. In some cases, adults target teens for grooming or exploitation, leveraging social media to initiate contact. The anonymity of the internet allows perpetrators to hide their identities, making it challenging to identify and stop them.

Research indicates that some teenagers who have been victims of doxing may, in turn, engage in doxing others. A study found that approximately 11% had participated in doxing behaviours. The study also noted that those who had experienced doxing themselves were more likely to disclose personal information about others, suggesting a potential cycle of retaliation or normalising of such behaviour.

Inside the mind of online stalkers and doxers

While Melanie thought she'd done everything right to protect herself from her stalker, things took a different turn for her when her stalker began posting her personal details online to scare and control her further. What started as stalking became something much more dangerous by exposing Melanie's private life to the public and putting her personal safety at risk.

Both stalking someone online and doxing their personal information online often come from the same place. These aren't just mean or rude actions; they are driven by deeper issues like obsession, jealousy, revenge, the need to control someone, or even the thrill of causing fear. When it gets to this level, things have escalated because the perpetrators haven't been able to get what they want.

It's important to understand these psychological motives because they can help you recognise warning signs early, protect yourself more effectively, and realise that the problem lies with the person's behaviour and has nothing to do with anything you have done.

What is the most important thing you need to know about cyberstalking and doxing?

These behaviours are not random. They come from a place of control, insecurity, or the need to hurt or dominate someone else, and they are never the victim's fault.

Obsession and fixation

One of the most common reasons people cyberstalk or dox others is obsession. This happens when someone becomes fixated on a person. The reasons are varied and can include that the victim is someone they have a crush on, used to date, admire, or even envy. Instead of respecting the other person's space, they feel the need to watch everything they do online. They might check their posts several times a day, save their photos, reply to every story they share, or monitor who they talk to.

Over time, this fixation can turn dangerous. The person may begin creating fake accounts to keep watching if you have blocked them, or may try to gather personal information, such as where you go to school or other parts of your life. What starts as interest becomes obsession, and for the person they are fixated on, it can feel invasive and frightening.

Control and power

Some people cyberstalk or dox others because they want to feel in charge. They may feel powerless in other parts of their lives and use online behaviour to dominate someone else. This is especially common in unhealthy or abusive relationships, where one person demands access to passwords, reads private messages, or uses apps to track someone's movements.

In these cases, doxing might be used as a threat: "If you leave me, I'll post your private life online, and they will see who you really are". Usually, it is used to punish someone who they feel refuses to conform to the behaviour they expect. The person doing it may convince themselves they're justified, but at its core, this is about trying to gain power by scaring, humiliating, or isolating you.

Revenge and jealousy

Revenge is a powerful motivator for online cyberstalking and doxing. Some people lash out after a breakup, argument, or rejection. Instead of dealing with their feelings in a healthy way, they try to hurt others by exposing private details, spreading lies, or encouraging others to attack them online.

Jealousy also plays a big role. If someone feels replaced, ignored, or threatened by your success or popularity, they may try to bring you down. Doxing becomes a way to attack your reputation through sharing your private location and embarrassing you in front of others to get even.

Insecurity and the need for validation

Some perpetrators are driven by low self-esteem or a desperate need to feel important. They may try to tear others down online to make themselves feel better. In group settings, doxing is sometimes done for peer approval based on what they feel is rewarded: by gaining status, impressing others, or being seen as powerful or popular.

In these cases, it becomes less about you and more about the cyberstalker or doxer's need for validation. They want to feel noticed, respected, or feared. Social media "likes", shares, and reactions can fuel this behaviour, making it seem like a game.

Narcissism and lack of empathy

Many people who stalk or dox others online show signs of narcissistic traits. This means they may believe they're more important than others, or that rules don't apply to them. They often lack empathy and don't consider or care about the emotional pain they cause.

Narcissistic behaviour can lead someone to feel entitled to someone else's attention or personal information. They might say things like "they owe me", or "I have a right to know what they're doing", even if the other person has clearly asked to be left alone. Their need for control or revenge can override any sense of right and wrong.

Sadism and the thrill of harm

Some people cyberstalk or dox others simply because they enjoy the chaos it causes. This is called sadistic behaviour. This is where some people take pleasure in someone else's fear, embarrassment, or pain. These individuals may not even know you personally; the thrill comes from wanting and receiving a reaction from you.

Sadistic doxing and trolling are especially common in toxic online communities, where cruelty is treated like entertainment. People are encouraged to expose others for fun, record their reactions, or push them until they break. This kind of abuse can make you feel devastated, and it often leaves lasting emotional scars.

Mental health struggles

In a small number of cases, online stalking and doxing are linked to mental health conditions, such as obsessive-compulsive behaviours, anxiety, paranoia, or delusional thinking. A person may believe they have a special connection with someone or misread online posts as secret messages.

While mental illness or poor emotional regulation can help explain some behaviours, it does not excuse them. No matter what the cause, violating someone's privacy, threatening them, or exposing their personal life online is never okay.

Understanding the motivations behind the person targeting Melanie helps reveal that these behaviours often come from underlying psychological issues, not from anything Melanie did wrong. Some people react in the wrong way when they don't get what they want. Cyberstalking and doxing might seem like problems that could only happen to other people, but the truth is that online anonymity makes it easier for people to target you without the usual offline world consequences. Many of these situations, including Melanie's, start from ordinary interactions, but when someone unstable or controlling doesn't manage feeling hurt, rejected, or jealous in a healthy way, they can twist into harmful or illegal behaviour that puts you at significant risk.

Check-in: What are the signs that you are being cyberstalked or doxed?

- ❐ Someone keeps contacting you after you've asked them to stop or blocked them
- ❐ They make new accounts or follow you across different apps or games
- ❐ They know personal details about you that you didn't share with them
- ❐ Someone threatens to share *or* actually shares your personal information (like your address, school, phone number, or private photos) online
- ❐ Your private details suddenly appear online or are sent to others without permission
- ❐ They try to scare, control, or silence you
- ❐ You feel watched, unsafe, anxious, or afraid online or offline

If you checked **one or more**, you are likely to be experiencing online stalking or doxing or both.

Staying one step ahead of being cyberstalked and doxed online

There are several steps Melanie could have taken to make it difficult for someone to gather information about her. You don't need to be technically savvy to take these steps. They are easy to follow, and you need to know how they can help you protect your privacy online. These steps are not set-and-forget; they should be habits. Protecting your information will protect you from cyberstalking and doxing.

1 Use unique and long passwords

Using the same password for all social media accounts may mean that if a password is leaked, discovered, compromised, or exposed in a data breach, an attacker has access to all the social media accounts that use that password, not just the account that was involved in the data breach, because the username is likely to be the same handle or email across the other social media accounts. For this reason, use a different password for every account.

Use a long password. Your password should be long (more than 12 characters) but easy to remember. Using pass phrases is an effective strategy because they tend to be long and easy to remember. For example, for a Snapchat password, one could use "Coolamononthegrow", which is the ad phrase for a nearby town (Note: Don't use this as your pass phrase). You can also use a password manager like 1Password, which can store all your complex passwords in your browser (if you turn on autofill). With a password manager, you only need to remember one password (the password to the password manager), but please note that password managers can also be hacked. If this happens, all your passwords, including those for your bank accounts, can be compromised.

2 Avoid using dictionary passwords

Any password in this list https://github.com/danielmiessler/SecLists/blob/master/Passwords/Software/john-the-ripper.txt can be cracked by an unskilled attacker in milliseconds – see below a screenshot of how fast John The Ripper password-cracking tool cracked the "trustno1" password, which is one of these dictionary passwords.

You can also sign up for data breach notification alerts for free at https://haveibeenpwned.com/. In addition to checking if your email has been exposed in a data breach, you can also get this website to notify you if your email has appeared in a data breach or surfaced on the dark web. If you have been notified that your password has been compromised, you should change it immediately.

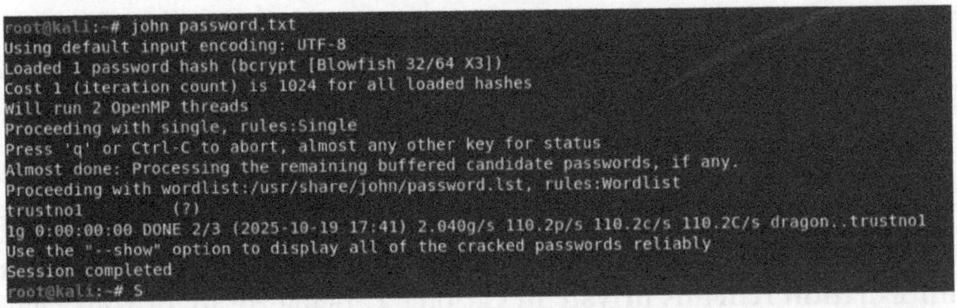

Read more information on recovering from and setting up data breach notifications in Chapter 6: Protecting Yourself from Sextortion and Image-Based Abuse

3 Enable multi-factor authentication (MFA)

With multi-factor authentication, even if someone got hold of your username and password, they would still need to get the code sent to your phone or generated by your authenticator app. Always keep MFA enabled, especially for your important accounts like banking, email, social media, and cloud storage. MFA via your authenticator app is more secure than MFA via text message, because unlike the code generated by your smartphone app, text messages can be spoofed or intercepted.

4 Adjust your privacy settings

Apps are designed to collect as much data about you as possible, and their default settings encourage constant data gathering. Check that the photos you take with your camera don't tag your location. Some apps tag your location in your posts without your knowledge. Turn off geotagging to disable location sharing and the "add to map" feature when posting photos on social media. Always check which apps on your smartphone have access to your location, microphone, and camera, and deny them access unless they absolutely need it.

Read more information on adjusting your location, microphone, and camera settings in Chapter 2: Smartphone Privacy, Security Settings, and Your Identifying Information

Likewise, always switch your public social media accounts to private mode and manage who can contact you, who can see your connections, your posts, and your personal information and contact details. The social media apps you use may connect to other apps; for example, the app you use to authenticate yourself to your social media accounts. Review these connected apps and if they don't need to have access to your social media accounts, revoke their access immediately. These connected apps not only collect your data without your knowledge but can also leak your data.

Read more information on adjusting your settings to ensure your information remains private in Chapter 1: Being Aware of Your Digital Footprint

5 Browse the web securely using freely available cybersecurity tools

Virtual private networks (VPNs) are great if you want to browse the web privately because not only do they hide your IP address, which can make it difficult for anyone to trace where you are connecting from (your actual IP address), but they also encrypt all your browsing traffic. If you have found yourself needing to access a public Wi-Fi, when you have run out of data and need to send an urgent message, then a VPN can give you that additional protection even if your data is sent to a non-secure website (http), that is, one that does not have the lock symbol (https[1]). Please note, though, that your IP address and all your encrypted data are not hidden from the VPN provider. The VPN provider can still see your data because they have decryption keys. Nevertheless, hiding your IP address, which is assigned to you by your internet service provider (ISP), is still worth doing because your actual IP address not only reveals your location, allowing attackers to track you, but also, using your IP address, attackers can hack into your machine if it is not secure.

Firewalls are your first line of defence against cyber-attacks. Firewalls block unwanted or suspicious incoming internet connections, so make sure your Windows Defender Firewall, on Windows machines, and macOS Firewall are always turned on.

The Firefox browser is known for its focus on security and privacy. You can use it for sensitive tasks like transacting with your bank over the web. You can configure it so it does not remember your browsing history and blocks trackers and third-party cookies. You should also be aware that when browsing in Incognito mode, the websites you visit can still see your IP address, the data you enter, your browser type, and location. All the Incognito mode does is isolate your browsing history from your regular profile by creating a temporary session for you in which your browsing history, cookies, and the search terms you type are not saved; so, if someone uses your device after you, they won't know what you did. But your ISP, and the owner of the network you used to browse the internet (work, school, home), can still see everything.

6 Remove metadata from your posts

The same tools you use to access the information you see online can be used to remove the hidden metadata from your social media posts. These tools can help you remove GPS coordinates, camera type, and timestamps. Removing the hidden metadata from the photos and videos you post to your social media accounts can stop stalkers and doxers from building a profile of you that details your movements across time and space.

> **Read more information on tools that can access your information online and remove hidden metadata can be found in** Chapter 9: How to Avoid Fake News and Online Misinformation

What to do if you are being cyberstalked and doxed online

You can imagine how distressing it would have been for Melanie to realise she was being stalked and doxed online. When someone targets you this way, it can feel overwhelming, scary, and out of your control, especially when your private life suddenly feels exposed or when you feel you are being watched. If this is happening to you, it's important to know that you're not alone, it's not your fault, and there are clear steps you can take to protect yourself and get support.

1 Stay calm and don't react publicly

If someone is stalking you online or posts your personal information (like your address, phone number, school, or photos), it's natural to feel scared or upset. But don't respond emotionally or publicly, as this can encourage them to keep going as they become validated by getting a response. Ensure you avoid replying to messages or posts and don't show any acknowledgement or emotional response online. Never engage or confront the stalker. Their goal is often to engage you to confirm that you are suffering from their actions.

2 Save and record everything

Even if it's upsetting and you just want it to stop, keeping a record is one of the strongest ways to protect yourself. Screenshots and notes help adults, platforms, or authorities understand what's happening and take action. Without proof, it can be harder to stop the person or get help.

If you have been cyberstalked or groomed:

- ☑ Take screenshots of messages, comments, posts, images, or threats
- ☑ Save usernames, profile links, email addresses, and account names
- ☑ Write down dates, times, and where it happened (apps, games, platforms)
- ☑ Keep copies of messages and profiles, even if they're deleted later
- ☑ Record any attempts to contact you across multiple platforms

- ☑ Note any offline behaviour (e.g., someone showing up near your home, school, or activities)

If possible, store this evidence in a safe place, such as a private folder, cloud storage, or with a trusted adult. You don't need to look at it often, and just knowing it's saved gives you options if you decide to report it later. Keeping records isn't about reliving what happened; it's about taking back control.

3 Lock down your online presence

Take steps straight away to protect your information and reduce your digital footprint. The goal is to make it harder for someone to track, contact, or target you.

- ☑ Change passwords to strong, unique ones
- ☑ Turn off location sharing on all apps
- ☑ Set accounts to private mode and log out of unfamiliar devices
- ☑ Turn on two-factor authentication
- ☑ Disable GPS tagging on posts and photos
- ☑ Remove your name from directories

Remember

If private or harmful info has been shared about you:

- Contact the platform using its reporting tools
- Describe what was posted, why it's wrong, and how it's harming you
- Ask websites to take down your phone number or address
- If it's a personal website, contact the web host

4 Block and report the person

Blocking and reporting sends a clear message and limits contact. Use each platform's tools to report doxing, threats, or impersonation. Ensure you report fake accounts. Most importantly, call the police if you're in physical danger.

Blocking and reporting are among the most important steps you can take. They prevent the person from contacting you directly and show the platform that their behaviour is not okay. Even if it feels uncomfortable or you're worried about making things worse, blocking does not cause someone to "win" as it protects you.

Use the reporting tools on each app, game, or platform to flag behaviour like harassment, threats, doxing, grooming, or impersonation. Platforms rely on reports to remove fake accounts, limit harmful users, and prevent them from targeting others. If the person keeps coming back under new usernames, report those accounts too.

These are serious forms of abuse and should be reported: Cyberstalking and doxing are *serious crimes*, with penalties including police charges, fines, and even jail. Sharing your address or phone number (without your permission) is illegal and can lead to criminal or civil action. Schools can take action too, including suspension, expulsion, and reporting the behaviour to police or child protection services.

5 Reach out for support

You don't need to face this alone. Talk to a trusted adult, such as a parent, caregiver, teacher, or counsellor. Let your friends and family know what's going on. Ask them not to engage with the stalker and to review their own privacy settings.

If the situation moves beyond the screen, for example, if someone threatens you, shares your personal information, pressures you to meet up, or tries to find you in real life, treat it as serious and urgent. Your safety comes first. Reach out to a trusted adult and contact local authorities if you feel at risk. Online harm can quickly become real-world danger, and getting help early is a strong and smart response, not an overreaction.

You should look up your government's available sources to report cyberstalking and doxing and receive support. Think about your offline safety too as online stalking can cross into the real world. Be mindful of who knows your location and routines.

Search online for "stalking helpline teens", "protection against stalking", or "reporting online stalking or doxing [add your country]".

Conclusion

Cyberstalking and doxing are growing online threats that can cause serious fear and distress, especially when someone's personal information is exposed. This chapter explored how cyberstalkers operate, why they target others, and the ways teens can protect their online presence. It also outlined practical steps for staying safe, supporting someone who has been targeted, and understanding the legal options and reporting tools available to address online harm. To protect yourself from these online harms, (1) use long and unique passwords, preferably passphrases, and use a different password for every account, (2) avoid using dictionary passwords, and (3) enable multi-factor authentication (MFA) for all important accounts. (4) Adjust your privacy settings to deny apps access to your location, microphone and camera, which will limit what others can see about you. (5) Browsing the web securely using freely available cybersecurity tools can protect your connection and identity, and (6) removing the metadata from your photos and videos, which can reveal your location, can keep your digital footprint private.

Key terms

- Cyberstalking
- Doxing (also Doxxing)
- Narcissistic behaviour
- Sadism
- Data breach
- Dictionary passwords
- Multi-factor authentication (MFA)
- Virtual private network (VPN)
- Cyber-attacks
- Firewalls

Note

1 The secure version of HTTP is actually "plain" HTTP sent over Transport Layer Security (TLS). HTTPS stands for Hypertext Transport Protocol Secure (HTTPS).

Bibliography

Anti-Defamation League. (2021). *Hate no game: Harassment and positive social experiences in online games 2021*. https://www.adl.org/resources/report/hate-no-game-harassment-and-positive-social-experiences-online-games-2021

Australian Bureau of Statistics. (2025, September 15). *Online safety*. https://www.abs.gov.au/statistics/measuring-what-matters/measuring-what-matters-themes-and-indicators/secure/online-safety

Carloss, T. (2024, June 24). *Man who traveled looking for girl who police say he cyberstalked, family speaks out to warn other parents*. News 5. https://www.news5cleveland.com/news/local-news/man-who-traveled-looking-for-girl-who-police-say-he-cyberstalked-family-speaks-out-to-warn-other-parents

Centers for Disease Control and Prevention. (2024). *Youth risk behavior survey data summary & trends report: 2013–2023*. U.S. Department of Health and Human Services. https://www.cdc.gov/yrbs/dstr/index.html

Chen, M., Cheung, A.S.Y., & Chan, K.L. (2019). Doxing: What adolescents look for and their intentions. *International Journal of Environmental Research and Public Health*, *16*(2), 218. https://doi.org/10.3390/ijerph16020218

CUNY. (n.d.). *Doxing*. https://www.cuny.edu/about/administration/offices/transformation/diversity-equity-and-inclusion-hub/doxing/

Cyber Helpline. (n.d.). *Dealing with cyberstalking*. https://www.thecyberhelpline.com/guides/cyber-stalking

Frontiers in Digital Child Safety Working Group. (2025). *Frontiers in digital child safety: Designing a child-centered digital environment that supports rights, agency, and well-being* (S. Cortesi & U. Gasser, Eds.). TUM Think Tank at the Munich School of Politics and Public Policy, Technical University of Munich; Berkman Klein Center for Internet & Society, Harvard University; Department of Communication and Media Research, University of Zurich.

Gitnux. (2026). *Cyber stalking statistics*. https://gitnux.org/cyber-stalking-statistics/

Harley, S. (2025). *Cyberstalking affects young people and gender minorities*. https://phys.org/news/2025-07-cyberstalking-faster-stalking-reveals.html

Janickyj, M., Blom, N., & Tanczer, L.M. (2025). Crime survey for England and Wales: Its predictors and victim/survivors' views on criminalisation. *The British Journal of Criminology, azaf064*. https://doi.org/10.1093/bjc/azaf064

Kapernick, K., & Moseley, A. (2024, May 15). *BTN high: Young people share experiences of being doxxed*. ABC News. https://www.abc.net.au/news/2024-05-15/btn-high-young-people-share-experiences-of-being-doxxed/103838534

Kim, M., Ellithorpe, M., & Burt, S.A. (2024). Anonymity and its role in digital aggression: A systematic review. *Aggression and Violent Behavior, 74*, 101856. https://doi.org/10.1016/j.avb.2023.101856

Law Reform Commission Victoria. (2022). *Responses to cyberstalking*. https://www.lawreform.vic.gov.au/publication/stalking-final-report/3-responses-to-cyberstalking/

McCall, M. (2024). *Cyberbullying statistics and legal overview*. https://www.findlaw.com/criminal/criminal-charges/cyberbullying-statistics.html

Moseley, A. (2025, July 25). *What to do if you've been doxxed*. ABC News. https://www.abc.net.au/btn/high/what-to-do-if-you-ve-been-doxxed/103847288

Office of the eSafety Commissioner. (2025, April 7). *Cyberstalking*. https://www.esafety.gov.au/key-topics/staying-safe/cyberstalking

Office of the eSafety Commissioner. (2026, March 13). *Gendered violence*. https://www.esafety.gov.au/key-topics/gendered-violence

Parliament of Australia. (2022, February 15). *eSafety Commissioner opening statement: Additional budget estimates 2021–22*. https://www.aph.gov.au/-/media/Estimates/ec/bud2122/Tabled_docs/esafety_commissioner_opening_statement.pdf

Perenc L. (2022). Psychopathic personality disorder and cybercriminality: An outline of the issue. *Current Issues in Personality Psychology, 10*(4), 253–264. https://doi.org/10.5114/cipp.2022.114205

Pew Research Center. (2022, December 15). *Teens and cyberbullying 2022*. https://www.pewresearch.org/internet/2022/12/15/teens-and-cyberbullying-2022/

Powell, A., Flynn, A., & Hindes, S. (2022). *Technology-facilitated abuse: National survey of Australian adults' experiences* (Research report, 12/2022). ANROWS.

Prall, D. (2026, February 26). *Cyberstalking statistics*. SafeHome. https://www.safehome.org/data/cyberstalking-statistics/

Scott, E. (2024, June 25). *Timothy Nielsen cyberstalking case involving girl and YouTube bodycam footage*. UNILAD. https://www.unilad.com/news/us-news/timothy-nielsen-cyberstalking-girl-youtube-bodycam-footage-844014-20240625

Shop, L. (2018, April 8). *New software by MIT, dubbed "Squad Box," hopes to combat cyberbullying*. ABC News. https://abcnews.go.com/Technology/software-mit-dubbed-squad-box-hopes-combat-cyberbullying/story?id=54304260

Silva Santos, I.L., Pimentel, C.E., & Mariano, T.E. (2023). Cyberstalking scale: development and relations with gender, FOMO and social media engagement. *Current psychology (New Brunswick, N.J.), 42*(6), 4802–4810. https://doi.org/10.1007/s12144-021-01823-3

Thomsen, E., Henderson, M., Moore, A., Price, N., & McGarrah, M.W. (2024). *Student reports of bullying: Results from the 2022 school crime supplement to the National Crime Victimization Survey* (NCES 2024–109rev). U.S. Department of Education. Washington, DC: National Center for Education Statistics. https://nces.ed.gov/pubsearch/pubsinfo.asp?pubid=2024109rev.

University of Maryland. (n.d.). *Doxing resources.* https://ogc.umd.edu/doxing

UNSW Newsroom. (2024, May 27). *More than 300 million child victims of online sexual abuse globally report.* https://www.unsw.edu.au/newsroom/news/2024/05/more-than-300-million-child-victims-of-online-sexual-abuse-globally-report

Vogels, E. (2021, January 13). *The state of online harassment.* Pew Research Center. https://www.pewresearch.org/internet/2021/01/13/the-state-of-online-harassment/

Walsh, W.A., Finkelhor, D., & Turner, H. (2025). Characteristics and dynamics of cyberstalking victimization among juveniles and young adults. *Violence Against Women, 31*(5), 1306–1327. https://doi. org/10.1177/10778012231225238

Zhang, W., Huang, S., Lam, L., Evans, R., & Zhu, C. (2022). Cyberbullying definitions and measurements in children and adolescents: Summarizing 20 years of global efforts. *Frontiers in Public Health, 10*, 1000504. https://doi.org/10.3389/fpubh.2022.1000504

6 Protecting yourself from sextortion and image-based abuse

As Zoe gently closed the car door, JoAnne, her mother, lowered the car window and affectionately yelled, "Where is my smile?" Turning her head towards her mum with a smile that drew a deep sigh from her, Zoe immediately turned to the sitting area below the school drop-off/pick-up area. As her mum drove off, Zoe noticed something unusual going on in the school as she slowly walked down the steps into the area. Instead of the lively scene she was used to in the morning, Zoe was greeted with a sombre atmosphere, in which students stood in small circles silently staring at their smartphones, quietly whispering to each other, and stealthily glancing at her. The girls' stares were more provocative. "What on earth is going on?" she asked, as she approached her two best friends, Sarah and Emily, who stood away from everyone else. The distressed looks on her besties' faces made Zoe feel even more anxious. "What happened? Tell me!" Sarah and Emily could not utter a word. After Zoe nervously begged for an answer, Emily handed Zoe her phone. Zoe froze. "What is this? What the hell is this? Who did this?" yelled Zoe. "Who did this?" she screamed. The students close by looked in her direction but pretended to be unconcerned. Putting her hand on her mouth, Zoe's reaction soon changed from utter shock to crying hysterically, and if it was not for Sarah, who helped her sit down on the bench, she would have fallen to the ground. Meanwhile, one of the boys came close to Emily and said, "Tell your friend not to be too upset; everyone knows these images were generated by AI. They are not real". Upon seeing her mother's car arrive, Zoe ran to the car. "What happened?" her mum asked as Zoe opened the door. "Just drive, mum, please," Zoe said. "Just drive." After driving for a few minutes, JoAnne pulled over by the side of the road and said to her daughter, "I am not going anywhere unless you tell me what happened". At first, Zoe could not tell her mother what happened, but when her mum insisted, Zoe showed her phone and mumbled that someone used an app to create

DOI: 10.4324/9781003681731-7

naked images of her and shared them on Snapchat. Sobbing uncontrollably, Zoe threw herself into her mother's arms. JoAnne gave her daughter a squeezy hug and then rushed to the nearest police station. The story continues ...

The escalating threat of sextortion and image-based abuse

Sextortion and image-based abuse (IBA) are serious online dangers that are becoming more common around the world. Sextortion happens when someone tricks or pressures you into sharing explicit photos or videos and then threatens to share them unless you do what they want. It might start as friendly, flirty, or even romantic, but it can quickly turn into blackmail. IBA is when someone shares or threatens to share your private or intimate images without your permission. This is often used to scare, control, or humiliate people.

Both these crimes can seriously affect your mental health, and many people stay quiet because they feel ashamed or afraid. But remember to protect yourself, and if something happens, it's not your fault, and help is always available.

What is the difference between sextortion and image-based abuse?

- **Sextortion** is online blackmail where perpetrators will encourage or force you to send explicit images or perform sexual acts on camera and demand money or more content under threats of exposure or harm. An innocent online connection can quickly become a dangerous trap.
- **Image-based abuse (IBA)** involves sharing or threatening to share intimate images without consent, whether originally shared voluntarily, altered, fake, or obtained deceitfully.

Who is at risk and who is targeting you?

Sextortion and IBA don't affect everyone the same way, and sadly, girls are more often targeted. Girls aged 15–17 are twice as likely as boys the same age to report being victims. LGBTQ+ teens are also at higher risk. Some studies show they are more than twice as likely to be targeted, often because the abuser threatens to "out" them.

But there's more to this. Even though girls are more likely to report sextortion or IBA, many boys keep quiet, often because of shame or pressure to "stay tough". This silence can be dangerous. International reports about sextortion incidents show that boys who experience sextortion are more likely to suffer alone and are also more likely to take their own lives after being blackmailed.

Most people who commit sextortion or IBA are men. Sometimes, the abuser is even a current or former partner, which means the victim may have once trusted them. Others use fake profiles or pretend to be someone else online. Some young men aged 18–24 are involved both as victims and perpetrators, which shows just how complicated and challenging this issue can be.

A study has revealed that many sextortion cases involving teens often involve much older men overseas, especially from countries like Nigeria, India, and Eastern Europe. These people use the anonymity of the internet to find and target teens on social media, gaming sites, or dating apps. They often pretend to be someone safe that you can trust, and think that being in a different country means the police cannot find them. They can work in groups or even as part of criminal gangs, and once they have a private photo, they demand more or ask for money, sometimes, in cryptocurrency or gift cards, to stay hidden. Because they're operating from outside the country, it can be hard to catch them, but law enforcement authorities always try to track and stop these networks.

A tragic story of how severe the consequences of sextortion are is that of 15-year-old Bryce Tate, who died by a self-inflicted gunshot wound just hours after being targeted in an online sextortion scheme. Bryce received a message from an unknown number and was contacted for about three hours before he died due to that sextortion attempt. Bryce's father said the scammer posed as a local 17-year-old girl and built trust using personal details of Bryce before asking for explicit images and cash. In the final minutes, Bryce was reportedly bombarded with numerous threatening messages, and his family claims the scammer encouraged him to take his life. Bryce's father described the scammer as exploiting his son's vulnerability.

Scams can be extremely targeted and traumatic

One of the fastest-growing threats facing teens is online sexual extortion (sextortion). Recent studies indicate that more than one in ten adolescents have experienced some form of sextortion, with many incidents occurring before the age of 16. In many cases, scammers first build trust through messaging apps or social media, then use threats, such as sharing private images or information, to demand money or more content. Globally, reports of online enticement and sextortion involving young people have increased dramatically in recent years, highlighting how quickly these threats are spreading.

A recent tragic case is of a teenage boy who died just hours after being targeted in an alleged online sextortion scam. The teen was contacted online by someone posing as a peer, who quickly manipulated him into sharing an intimate image. The scammer then threatened to distribute the image to his family and social media contacts unless money was paid. Despite the intense pressure and fear created by these threats, the teen had little time to process what was happening or seek help. The case highlights the severe psychological impact sextortion can have on young people, particularly when scammers use shame, urgency, and isolation to overwhelm victims.

Teenagers are also regularly exposed to online abuse, impersonation, and manipulation, even when they don't directly engage with scammers. Surveys show that over half of teens have encountered cyberbullying, threats, or harassment online, while many others report exposure to misinformation or extremist content. These experiences can blur the line between what is safe and unsafe online, making it harder to recognise when a situation is becoming risky.

AI-generated nudes and deepfakes

Lately, there's been a scary rise in cases where teens are being targeted with AI-generated explicit images. These images are created using "Nudify" apps that strip clothing from real photos to make fake nudes. These fake images are then used to bully, blackmail, or harass victims. Deepfake sexualised videos are also on the rise. One good quality image is all that these AI deepfake apps require to create a deepfake sexualised video of someone, and it costs nothing.

One heartbreaking story is about a 16-year-old boy named Elijah Heacock from the United States. He tragically died by suicide after being targeted in an online sextortion scam involving AI-generated nude photos of himself. He received anonymous texts with these fake images and threats to release them unless he paid a ransom.

> **Did you know?** Over 40% of victims targeted with these digital deepfakes never even met their abusers in person. Some of these crimes are linked to global digital cults and organised crime networks, causing severe psychological impacts, including cases of suicide.

Because of the rise in AI-generated explicit content, laws are being enacted to protect people. In the United States, the "Take It Down Act" was passed to combat nonconsensual intimate imagery, including AI-generated deepfake nudes. This law makes it illegal to post such content without consent and requires online platforms to remove reported content within 48 hours. Australia has similar protections. Creating, sharing, or threatening to share intimate images, including AI-generated or digitally altered images, without consent is a crime under Australian law. These offences can carry serious penalties, including fines and prison time. These laws are a big step towards protecting individuals from the harms of AI-generated sexual abuse.

Concerning trends and worrying psychological insights

Zoe's experience with AI-generated images being created and shared without her consent is becoming more common. In 2025, such cases have more than doubled, with 80% of the victims being female. What makes cases like Zoe's especially alarming is not just the images themselves, but the serious psychological impact they can have when experiencing something so hurtful. Behind the growing numbers of sextortion and IBA cases are patterns of manipulation, fear, and trauma that affect your mental health in deep ways. By understanding these concerning trends and the tactics predators use, you can better protect yourself and support others who may have also experienced the same thing.

You might trust someone, but that doesn't mean it's safe to send nudes

A lot of teens are pressured into sending explicit photos of themselves because they think they're in a close relationship, or that the other person truly cares about them. But many cases of sextortion and IBA start with images that the victim sent themselves, often during private chats or sexting with someone they thought was a close friend or romantic partner.

Even if you feel like you can trust someone now, things can change, and once an image is sent, you can't control where it ends up. That's why it's so important to never send nudes, no matter how much pressure you're under or how "safe" it might feel at the time.

Some people try to shame victims by saying "they sent the photo themselves", but that's not fair or true. Just because someone trusted the wrong person doesn't mean they deserved what happened. No one should ever be blamed for being manipulated, and help is always available if you've been targeted.

Sextortion doesn't always happen slowly

You might think you'd be able to spot someone grooming you over time, but scammers and bots can strike within minutes of messaging you. These predators often use pre-written scripts and threats, and once they get what they want (or don't), they quickly move on to their next target.

A lot of these scams aren't even about sex; they're about money. Many are run by criminal networks overseas that treat sextortion like a business. They're doing it for profit, and they're ruthless. Once they have a photo or piece of information, they'll do anything to make you feel scared, ashamed, and trapped just so you'll pay up or send more.

It's important to know this has nothing to do with you doing something "wrong". It's a scam, and they're counting on fear to keep you quiet. You are not alone, and there are people who can help.

Read more information on online grooming, which is a psychological aspect of sextortion and IBA predators: Chapter 7: Recognising and Responding to Catfishing and Online Grooming

It can happen offline by people you once trusted

A boyfriend or girlfriend might threaten to share private photos to control you or get their way. They might use these threats during breakups, accuse you of cheating, or try to pressure you into doing things you don't want to do. This is a type of digital abuse and control, similar to how adults can be abusive in relationships.

When a partner or ex-partner uses private images to hurt or control someone, it often comes from emotional "dysregulation", meaning they struggle to manage intense feelings like anger, jealousy, or rejection. A breakup, argument, or loss of control can feel overwhelming to them, and instead of coping in healthy ways, they react impulsively. Sharing or threatening to share images becomes a way to release their distress and regain a sense of power.

For some people, this behaviour is linked to entitlement and objectification. They may see their partner less as a person and more as something that belongs to them. This makes it easier for them to ignore empathy and boundaries. In these cases, the images are no longer about intimacy; they are now tools. Psychological research shows that when empathy drops and entitlement rises, people are more likely to justify harmful actions, even towards someone they once claimed to care about.

There can also be elements of narcissism or fragile self-esteem. If someone's self-worth depends on feeling admired or in control, rejection can feel like an attack on their identity. Rather than feeling sadness or grief, they may experience rage or humiliation and try to "win" by causing harm. This doesn't mean they are always violent people, but it does mean they lack the emotional skills to handle loss without hurting others.

Online environments also reduce accountability and empathy due to the disinhibition they foster, leading people to behave in ways they wouldn't in real-life, face-to-face interactions. When abuse happens through screens, people are more likely to detach from the real impact of their actions. This psychological distance can make it easier for someone to do things online that they might never do face-to-face. That's why IBA can escalate quickly after a breakup or conflict.

Read more information on why people act differently online due to disinhibition in Chapter 4: Becoming Resilient to Cyberbullying and Trolling

Gaming and social platforms are predator playgrounds

Sextortion is happening everywhere. While Instagram and Snapchat are still common platforms for sharing photos, a lot of sextortion is now happening on platforms that feel more private or less watched, like Discord, TikTok, Kik, WhatsApp, and even chat features in games like Roblox, Fortnite, or Xbox Live. These places might seem fun and harmless, but they can also give predators the chance to build fake relationships with you through chatting, playing games, or pretending to be your friend. Predators use these platforms because of the large number of teens playing games, and because they are less experienced than adults in recognising grooming.

It's important to remember that the person on the other end might not be who they say they are, no matter how friendly they seem or how many photos they've shared. Anyone can fake a profile or copy someone else's pictures.

Always trust your instincts and be careful who you trust online. Never feel pressured to share anything personal or private.

Some predators are now using advanced tech to trick you

They might use AI-generated avatars or deepfake faces to pretend they're someone your age, someone cool, or someone you might be attracted to. Some even create fake profiles that look like they belong to popular classmates, using stolen photos or realistic AI-generated pictures to make it all seem real.

This is done to gain your trust, so you'll feel safe chatting or even sharing something private. But it's all fake. Some predators even use voice-changing apps or AI video tools to look and sound convincing on live video calls, but they're not who they claim to be.

If something feels off, trust your gut. No matter how real someone seems online, always be careful and don't share anything private or personal because once it's out there, it's out of your control.

Extortion can involve multiple demands

Predators often don't stop after getting one photo or video. They'll pressure you to send more, ask for videos, or even try to get you to do things live on a webcam. What starts as one message can turn into days, weeks, or even months of harassment.

In many cases, it doesn't end with threats and turns into blackmail for money. They might say, "Pay me, or I'll send this to your friends or family". It's scary, and it's meant to make you feel trapped.

People who do this kind of abuse often mess with your head on purpose

Predators use manipulation tactics that are a lot like what domestic abusers use. They try to isolate you, make you feel ashamed, or say things to make you feel guilty, like it's somehow all your fault. They might threaten to ruin your reputation or say, "You trusted me, so now you have to do what I say".

Even though IBA happens a lot, many teens don't speak up about it.

Despite the scale, IBA remains heavily under-reported. Many teens don't come forward because:

- ☑ They're scared their parents, caregivers, or school might punish them
- ☑ They feel ashamed or think it's their fault

- ☑ They don't realise what's happened is against the law, and people can help them
- ☑ They don't know where to go for help

Some people might not believe them, make fun of them, or blame them for what happened. Girls often get slut-shamed, while boys might be teased or ridiculed for "letting it happen". This is called secondary harm, and it's unfair, and no one deserves to be treated like that.

Zoe's story shows how quickly sextortion and IBA can turn a person's world upside down, from trust and friendship to fear and isolation. But while these experiences can feel overwhelming, it's important to be vigilant in how you protect yourself online. Similar to Zoe's situation, it is important to understand how quickly sextortion and IBA can happen based on how you are psychologically targeted online, even without you sharing anything yourself. That's why knowing what steps to take to protect yourself is important.

Check-in: Not all sextortion or image-based abuse looks obvious. In some cases, it happens gradually or quietly, making it harder to recognise. Use the list below to check whether you might be experiencing it:

- ☐ Someone is threatening to share photos, videos, or screenshots of you
- ☐ You hear that someone with whom you shared private photos is showing them to others
- ☐ You're being pressured to send more images, videos, or do things on a webcam
- ☐ They demand money, gift cards, crypto, or favours to "keep quiet"
- ☐ A partner jokes about "leaking" photos or reminds you they still have them, or says they will use them if you ever breakup with them
- ☐ They get angry if you ask for photos to be deleted and say it's your fault, or try to shame you for trusting them
- ☐ You feel scared, trapped, or panicked, like you have no way out
- ☐ They rush you, using urgency ("act now or I'll send this")
- ☐ You're afraid to say no because they have pictures or videos of you
- ☐ You're told not to tell anyone, especially parents, caregivers or teachers
- ☐ Images of you (real or AI-generated) are shared without your consent

If you recognised yourself in any of these signs, please tell a trusted adult as soon as possible. There is support, and there are safe ways to make this stop. What's happening to you is not okay or legal.

How attackers, predators, or perpetrators use technology to obtain and share abusive content

While perpetrators of sextortion and IBA use deception to lure their victims, they also rely heavily on technology to gain trust and access personal images. This can include fake profiles, stolen photos, AI-generated faces, or pretending to be someone you already know. In Zoe's case, she never shared any explicit images at all. Instead, images were created using AI from photos she had already posted online and then circulated by others. This shows that perpetrators don't need your consent or participation to cause harm when they can leverage technology to help them.

1 Nearly all cases involve fake profiles

If you receive an invite from a social media profile claiming to be your friend or a friend of a friend or someone from school, and you suspect they like you (e.g., a crush), don't immediately accept the invite. Instead, take the following steps to reduce any risks:

1 First, look up their profile. See who is connected to this profile. If your other friends, or the people you know from school who you would expect to be their friends, are not listed as connections, then this profile is likely to be fake.

2 Second, verify the profile is genuine and that the claim about your relationship to them is real:

- Don't ask them for their phone number, but if you already have their number in your contacts, call them or text them.
- If you don't have their number, you can talk to them in person in a public setting, like a school ground, "Hey, thanks for the Snapchat invite".
- It may be awkward for you and the person you asked if they are not the one who sent you the invite, but you are safer for it. **In this case, reject the invite without hesitation.**

2 They usually start with compliments, offers, or by trying to gain your trust

Once you accept their invitation, they may resort to other deceptive tactics like complimenting you, admiring things you do, giving you game credits, expressing affection towards you, or even promising to give you a good opportunity, like a job, modelling, or playing for a sports club, so you can trust them. Once they feel that you trust them, they will ask you to send them a photo of you; and once you send them one photo, they may threaten you to share it, unless you send them more photos or send them money.

3 They will often try to take you to apps or platforms where interactions can't be traced

They may even get you to continue communicating with them via an encrypted app, such as Telegram. The use of an encrypted app can make it extremely hard for law enforcement authorities to track the attackers, especially if they use other anonymisation tools like TOR. To get you to send them money, attackers will send you detailed and easy-to-follow instructions on how to deposit the money into a crypto ATM. These machines are often located in shopping malls and petrol stations and behave similarly to regular bank ATMs. The attackers will receive the money in cryptocurrency because it is difficult to trace.

4 They will try to hack your email and password to get access to private photos or videos

Sextortionists and IBAs often don't need to deceive you at all to obtain your private photos and videos. Your private photos and videos can be obtained through hacking into your social media accounts. There have been numerous cyber-attacks in recent years that resulted in data breaches. Large healthcare, health insurance, telecommunications, and financial services organisations, as well as airlines, have been successfully targeted and experienced cyber-attacks that resulted in data breaches. One implication of these cyber-attacks is that your credentials are likely to be either made accessible by cyber criminals in plaintext via the dark web or that unskilled hackers can purchase them from the cyber criminals as part of a wholesale sale of passwords.

You can check if your email has been implicated (compromised) in a data breach incident by entering it in the search box of this website: https://haveibeenpwned.com/, which is curated by Troy Hunt, a trusted Australian cybersecurity researcher. If you use the same username and passwords across multiple social media platforms, then you just made it easier for attackers to target you. Also, if you use a commonly used password, like "trustno1", then an attacker needs only milliseconds to crack your password using a free tool like John The Ripper. If your password appears in this list of more than 3,000 dictionary passwords https://github.com/danielmiessler/SecLists/blob/master/Passwords/Software/john-the-ripper.txt, then you need to change it immediately and across all sites in which your password is used because any freely available software can crack any of these passwords in no time. Similarly, if you use a short password, any easy-to-use, freely available online brute-force software can crack it. The longer the password, the more secure it is.

In addition to retrieving your private photos and videos by hacking into your social media account, having compromised your account's credentials, attackers can also obtain them through cyber scams. Attackers can use phishing attacks that can socially engineer you to click on a link sent to you via a spoofed SMS message to reveal your password. Once attackers have access to your social media account, they can obtain any sensitive photos or videos of you.

Read more information on phishing attacks and how they use links in Chapter 3: Protecting Your Online Privacy and Mitigating Cybersecurity Threats

5 They will use the information they obtained to blackmail you

Attackers can also try to compromise your phone or your Apple iCloud. Once attackers succeed in retrieving your sensitive photos and videos, there is nothing that can stop them from blackmailing you (sextortion). If the photos the attackers retrieved are not explicit, as highlighted above, they can just use any deepfake algorithmic AI agent to generate a sexually explicit image of you that can show you in a situation you were never involved with in 3D. It can appear lifelike or real, even though they are completely fake. For the extortion to be effective, attackers need to know more about you. For example, they need to know who your friends are, especially your school friends; this can help guarantee your compliance to avoid embarrassment. To do this, they can simply scour your list of social media connections. It is also easy for them to know your physical location. Did you know that your smartphone camera associates the photos you take with the time and location where you took them? This metadata is important to attackers because when blackmailing you, they can say to you, this is where you live or this is the school you go to, to scare you. Make sure you disable this feature in your phone when taking selfies and only post photos taken by your phone after you strip the photo of this metadata, especially the location.

6 Platforms are using AI to help combat this abuse

The good news is that social media platforms are now beginning to use AI for good, including as a countermeasure to deepfake algorithmic AI agents. In this context, AI can now be used to detect and prevent sextortion and IBA. AI tools can flag images as explicit. Instagram, for example, can blur explicit photos (photos that contain nudity) that are sent privately via a direct message on the recipient's device.

AI tools can also scan social media platforms for uploaded sexual content, block it, hide it, or remove such content. Tech giants are now also beginning to watermark AI generated content (embed a hidden message) to make it clear that an image or video is not original or one that was created by a human. An example of this is Google SynthID. While not all AI agents attach a detectable signature to the images they create, the effort to distinguish fake from real is gaining momentum.

Another technology being used for good in this context is encryption. When a victim of sextortion or IBA registers an image or a video with a service like StopNCII.org, the image is given a hash (a digital fingerprint). Social media platforms can scan the image against the registered one; if a match is found, it will delete it. This helps prevent the image from being copied and spread to other social media platforms. So, if you come across an image of yourself that you don't approve of, register it.

Social media platforms crawl their networks for sexual content, and in addition to active monitoring, they are compelled by law, at least in the United States, the United Kingdom, the European Union, and Australia, to act swiftly to takedown notices. When a victim of sextortion or IBA submits a takedown request, the social media platform has a legal obligation to remove the content.

Social media platforms are also collaborating in this space by sharing information about sexual predator accounts, so they don't move from one platform to another when discovered. To avoid costly lawsuits, several social media platforms are beginning to strengthen the security settings for children's accounts; for example, by setting them to private rather than public mode and by blocking unknown contacts from sending direct messages (DM-ing).

What to do if you've been targeted by sextortion or image-based abuse

When Zoe found out that fake images of her were circulating online, she felt shocked and powerless, but she had many options to take control back and protect herself. Zoe never imagined she'd need help after discovering AI-generated images of herself being shared, yet knowing what to do made a huge difference in stopping the harm.

1 Don't give in to their demands

If someone is threatening you or trying to blackmail you for money or more pictures, don't reply or send anything. Stop all contact and don't try to negotiate with them. Giving in doesn't make the problem go away, and it usually makes them demand more. Every time you respond, you show them they can control you. Even if they promise to stop, they're likely to keep asking.

If you are being blackmailed:

- ✓ Do not pay or give in to their demands, as paying does not guarantee they will stop.
- ✓ Save all evidence and keep every message, email, and screenshot, even if it's upsetting.
- ✓ Report to the police straight away, and the sooner they know, the sooner they can act.
- ✓ Reach out for support and talk to a trusted adult, friend, or support service for emotional help.

2 Keep proof of everything

Save every piece of evidence, including messages, emails, texts, chat logs, and any images or videos sent to you. Take clear screenshots that show usernames, dates, and times. If the threats are happening in apps where messages can disappear, take screenshots immediately. Don't delete anything, even if it's upsetting to look at, as these records are often the strongest proof to identify the offender and stop them. Keeping this evidence will also help police, lawyers, or online safety organisations take action in cases of sextortion or IBA. This information can help stop the person and support you if you need to report it.

3 Block and protect your account

Once you've saved all the evidence after realising someone is threatening, blackmailing, or sharing your private images, cut off their ability to contact you. Blocking them stops the harassment and gives you breathing space. Reporting them to the platform, the police, or a helpline helps hold them accountable and can prevent them from targeting others. Even if you're scared or embarrassed, remember you are not alone, and there are people who can help you get through this. It is important to stop all contact immediately, regardless of any threats or warnings. Ensure that you:

- ☑ Block the person on all platforms, apps, and phone numbers they are using to contact you
- ☑ Report their account to the social media site, messaging app, or gaming platform, as they can remove their profile and stop further abuse
- ☑ Check your social media privacy settings and make sure your accounts are secure
- ☑ Be wary of any new friend requests trying to message you, and validate profiles you don't know

You might trust someone today, but people change, and relationships can end. After a breakup, someone can act in ways you never expected, and you can't control what they do with private photos or videos of you once they have been sent. They can be shared, faked with AI, or used to threaten you. If you do choose to share images and put yourself at risk, never include your face or anything that can identify you; even your voice can be used to recognise you in videos by AI tools.

4 Get help from people you trust and support services

Talk to a parent, caregiver, teacher, school counsellor, or another trusted adult. There are people and organisations that know how to help you if you're dealing with sextortion or IBA. You don't have to handle this alone, so always reach out to trusted support services in your country or online. Most countries have:

- ☑ Helplines you can call or text for free, providing confidential advice and support
- ☑ Online specialised free chat services where you can talk to someone safely and privately
- ☑ Government resources for reporting abuse and removing harmful content from the internet
- ☑ Counsellors and specialists who understand what you're going through

You can also ask a trusted adult, like a teacher or school counsellor, to help you find the right support.

Search online for "[Your country] youth helpline"; "[Your country] cyber-safety support; teen sextortion helpline"

5 Tell the police

Sextortion and IBA are crimes. It is important to report it to the police and share the proof you have. Police have specialised training in dealing with these types of offences and can guide you through the process, prioritising your safety and well-being. When you make a report, you're not only standing up for yourself, but you're also helping prevent the same person from harming other people.

To make the process easier:

- Bring all the proof you have – save and provide screenshots, messages, emails, images, usernames, and any details about when and how you were contacted.
- Write down a timeline of events – this helps police understand what happened and when.

Important information that teens need to know about the law:

✓ Many teens don't know that even consensual sexting can be illegal if minors are involved.
✓ Possessing, sharing, or threatening to share intimate images, even if you created them, may carry serious criminal penalties.
✓ You can often report anonymously and ask for content to be removed through takedown services.

6 Look after yourself

This is really tough, and it's okay to feel upset. Talking to a counsellor or someone who understands can help you feel better and provide you with the support you need during this difficult time.

Remember

✓ This is NOT your fault
✓ Asking for help is brave, and there are people ready to support you
✓ The sooner you act, the better chance you have of stopping the abuse

Search online for "image-based abuse helpline teens"; "protection against sextortion"; or "reporting image-based abuse or sextortion [add your city]"

Conclusion

Sextortion is a growing threat where young people are blackmailed using explicit images they shared with other people who they thought they could trust. This chapter explained the psychological manipulation tactics used by perpetrators and how teens can recognise warning signs before victimisation occurs. It also addressed IBA, outlining legal consequences and resources available for victims. Attackers can use psychological manipulation techniques like social engineering to trick you into sending them intimate images of yourself. They can also hack into your social media account or obtain your login details from the dark web. Once they have accessed your photos, they can use them to create deepfakes of a sexual nature. Using the metadata in your photos, such as location, they can threaten to share your intimate images with others unless you comply with their requests. There are several steps you can take to protect yourself from sextortion and IBA. These include always verifying the account/profile that sent you a social media invite; never send a nude photo of yourself to anyone, always use strong passwords, and never click on a link in an SMS message. There is hope when it comes to combating these crimes. Social media platforms, AI agent developers, and governments are trying to contain the threat posed by these cyber crimes. But you need to do your bit to stay safe online.

Key terms

- Sextortion
- Image-based abuse (IBA)
- Sexting
- Nudify
- Deepfakes
- Nonconsensual
- Encrypted
- Cyber-attack
- Hacking
- DM-ing
- Encryption

Bibliography

Baker, K. (2025, June 9). *Teen was blackmailed with A.I.-generated nude photo of himself. Then he died by suicide.* People. https://people.com/teen-blackmailed-fake-nude-photo-sextortion-scam-suicide-11750620

Bureau Report. (2025, June 3). *AFP helps crack global sextortion ring linked to teen suicides.* The Australia Today. https://www.theaustraliatoday.com.au/afp-helps-crack-global-sextortion-ring-linked-to-teen-suicides/

Cooper, A. (2024, December 15). *Schools face a new threat: "nudify" sites that use AI to create realistic, revealing images of classmates.* CBS News. https://www.cbsnews.com/news/schools-face-new-threat-nudify-sites-use-ai-create-realistic-revealing-images-60-minutes-transcript/

Digby Werthmuller, D., & Rix, E. (2025, October 17). *Deepfake image-based abuse happening at least once a week in schools, eSafety data shows.* ABC News. https://www.abc.net.au/news/2025-10-17/deepfake-image-based-abuse-doubles-across-australia/105905152

eSafety Commissioner. (2017). *Image-based abuse qualitative research summary*, Canberra: Australian Government.

eSafety Commissioner. (2019). *Understanding the attitudes and motivations of adults who engage in image-based abuse.* Australian Government. https://www.esafety.gov.au/sites/default/files/2019-10/Research_Report_IBA_Perp_Motivations.pdf

eSafety Commissioner. (2024, December 23). *FAQ about image based abuse.* Australian Government. https://www.esafety.gov.au/key-topics/image-based-abuse/faq-about-image-based-abuse

eSafety Commissioner. (2025, December 16). *Online risks for women.* Australian Government. https://www.esafety.gov.au/women/online-risks-for-women

Federal Bureau of Investigation. (2024). *2023 internet crime report released.* https://www.ic3.gov/AnnualReport/Reports/2023_IC3Report.pdf

Forester, M. (2025, March 13). *Death of Kentucky teen sparks investigation into possible sextortion scheme.* ABC News. https://abcnews.com/US/death-kentucky-teen-sparks-investigation-sextortion-scheme/story?id=119709205

Giannini, D. (2024, June 11). *Young males are a top target for online sexual extortion: New study finds.* Herald Sun. https://www.heraldsun.com.au/truecrimeaustralia/police-courts-victoria/young-males-have-become-a-top-target-for-online-sexual-extortion-new-study-finds/news-story/60d2a17b56d50c1a43cd0cda2a9a51ef

Grant, J.I. (2017). Future leaders standing up to online abuse. *eSafety Commissioner.* https://www.esafety.gov.au/newsroom/blogs/future-leaders-standing-up-to-online-abuse

Henry, N., & Umbach, R. (2024). Sextortion: Understanding online sexual extortion. *Computers in Human Behavior, 158.* https://doi.org/10.1016/j.chb.2024.108298

Jargon, J. (2025, June 7). *'Sextortion' scams involving Apple Messages ended in tragedy for these boys.* The Wall Street Journal. https://www.wsj.com/tech/personal-tech/sextortion-scam-teens-apple-imessage-app-159e82a8

Killion, V.L. (2025, May 20). *The TAKE IT DOWN Act: A federal law prohibiting the nonconsensual publication of intimate images* (CRS Legal Sidebar LSB11314). Congressional Research Service. https://www.congress.gov/crs-product/LSB11314

Long, C. (2023, May 25). *Reports of sextortion triple in first quarter of 2023, with young men most at risk.* ABC News. https://www.abc.net.au/news/2023-05-25/instagram-snapchat-most-used-sextortion-esafety-commissioner/102388824

Milmo, D., & Brooks, L. (2025, March 9). *Children in UK as young as 11 targeted by sextortion criminals, data reveals.* The Guardian. https://www.theguardian.com/uk-news/2025/mar/09/children-in-uk-as-young-as-11-targeted-by-sextortion-criminals-data-reveals

Moore, C. (2025, December 10). *Teen dies 3 hours after being targeted in alleged 'sextortion' scam.* News.com.au. https://www.news.com.au/lifestyle/real-life/news-life/teen-dies-just-3-hours-after-being-targeted-in-alleged-sextortion-scam/news-story/6c75e3676f7f1a6a0151dbd9ae95760e

Office of the eSafety Commissioner. (2017). *Image-based abuse national survey: Summary report*, Canberra: Australian Government.

Office of the eSafety Commissioner. (2017). *Image-based abuse: Prevalence and pathways.* https://www.esafety.gov.au/research/image-based-abuse/prevalence-pathways

Parliament of Australia. (2024). *Bills Digest No. 81 2023–24 (bd2324a/24bd081).* https://www.aph.gov.au/Parliamentary_Business/Bills_Legislation/bd/bd2324a/24bd081

Patchin, J.W., & Hinduja, S. (2024). The nature and extent of youth sextortion: Legal implications and directions for future research. *Computers in Human Behavior.* https://www.sciencedirect.com/science/article/pii/S0747563224001663

Richter, R. (2025, December 10). *Promising student, 15, dead just hours after being swept up in international sextortion scheme targeting American teens.* Daily Mail. https://www.dailymail.com/news/article-15368331/teen-sextortion-scheme-suicide-america-west-virginia.html

RMIT University. (2024, June 11). *One in seven adults have experienced someone threaten to share their intimate images: Research.* https://www.rmit.edu.au/news/all-news/2024/june/sextortion

Teunissen, C., Cahill, M., Napier, S., Cubitt, T., Boxall, H., & Brown, R. (2024). Sexual exploitation of children on dating platforms and experiences of revictimisation as an adult. *Trends & Issues in Crime and Criminal Justice* no. 697, Canberra: Australian Institute of Criminology. https://doi.org/10.52922/ti77482

Thorn. (2023, June). *LGBTQ+ youth perspectives: How LGBTQ+ youth are navigating online risks.* https://info.thorn.org/hubfs/Research/Thorn_LGBTQ%2BYouthPerspectives_June2023_FNL.pdf

UNICEF Australia. (n.d.). *Self-harm and young people.* https://www.unicef.org.au/parent-teacher-resources/parent-and-teacher-mental-wellbeing/self-harm-young-people

Westgarth, G. (2025, May). *Teen's legacy continues after cruel sextortion scam claimed his life.* 9News. https://9now.nine.com.au/a-current-affair/teens-legacy-continues-after-cruel-sextortion-scam-claimed-his-life/36a81217-0e2c-405b-a54b-b303838291fe

Wolbers, H., Cubitt, T., Napier, S., Cahill, M., Nicholas, M., Burton, M., & Giunta, K. (2025). Sexual extortion of Australian adolescents: Results from a national survey. *Trends & Issues in Crime and Criminal Justice* no. 712, Canberra: Australian Institute of Criminology. https://doi.org/10.52922/ti77819

7 Recognising and responding to catfishing and online grooming

"Coming or what?" Liz's mum, Kate, shouted angrily as she walked towards Liz's room, to which Liz responded, "I told you I am not hungry." "What on earth did you do to yourself?" Kate asked, with her hand on her mouth, in utter shock. "Nothing, I am fine," 13-year-old Liz replied. "Go away, you are annoying," she continued in a shaken voice. "Did you shave off your eyebrows and your eyelashes?" Kate asked. "But why? Are you out of your mind?" Kate's voice grew visibly irritated. "It is fine, mum, it is fine," Liz responded. "But why?" Kate insisted. "How are you going to go to school like that? Did you actually stop for a second and think about that?" Kate roared in a commanding tone. Just as she uttered the words "It is not a biggie" while scrolling on her phone, Liz recognised herself in the TikTok compilation video, hashtagged 'Idiots taking the shaving off eyebrows and eyelashes challenge'. Liz kicked her mum out of the room, slammed the door shut, and directly text-chatted her evil friend. "You posted the video I sent you on TikTok! Why did you do that?" Liz's first message read. "You are mean," she added, followed by "You tricked me" and "I hate you." No response received. Meanwhile, her mum's attempt to enter Liz's room to comfort her daughter failed. Liz wanted to be alone. She is shocked and can't believe this has actually happened to her. She wished she were dead. She wanted to go to sleep so that she could wake up and discover it was just a nightmare that she had, but she couldn't fall asleep. The thought of everyone at school laughing at her is playing on her mind. "This is the worst day in my life," Liz thought to herself, as she cried in silence. She was not sure what she felt. Did she feel ashamed, embarrassed or humiliated, or all of the above? In the meantime, her mum continued to check on her.

***

After three days of sniffling in her room and missing school, Liz finally confessed to her mum that a guy she thought of as her best friend in Roblox challenged her to shave off her eyebrows and eyelashes, so she did. Before this revelation, her mum had never even heard of Roblox, so to protect her daughter from future attacks like these, Kate got Liz to help her create a

DOI: 10.4324/9781003681731-8

Roblox account and link it to her daughter's account. From her account, Kate clicked on Settings, and from there she clicked on Parental Controls. Having located the Roblox connection who manipulated her daughter into filming herself shaving off her eyebrows and eyelashes, Kate not only blocked this connection, preventing him from ever contacting her daughter, but also reported him, effectively filing a complaint against that user. Kate also changed the content maturity and label levels to one appropriate for her daughter's age. Liz put an incorrect age in the app, so her mum entered her correct age and also reduced her screentime.

The hidden dangers behind trusting others online

Catfishing is when someone pretends to be someone else online, usually by using fake photos, names, ages, or even stolen identities to trick others. They might pretend to be a teen to get closer to other teens. Sometimes it's for attention or money, but other times it can lead to much more dangerous behaviour. Catfishers might act like they want to be your friend or boyfriend/girlfriend, but everything they say is a lie. Their goal is to gain your trust, keep you talking, and manipulate you. Some even steal real identities by gaining trust and accessing photos, dates of birth, and locations to make their fake profiles seem more convincing.

Recent data shows that 23% of teens aged 13–17 have been contacted by someone who later turned out to be lying about who they were. In fact, 78% of teens say they regularly encounter fake profiles on platforms like Instagram, Snapchat, and Facebook, where 81% of all catfishing incidents take place. Social media apps with disappearing messages, like Snapchat, are especially risky and are used in nearly half of the reported grooming cases. These scams often last three to six months before the truth comes out, and nearly 60% of victims say it made them more cautious or mistrustful of others online.

What are catfishing and grooming?

Catfishing: The term "catfishing" originates from a 2010 documentary film in which Nev Schulman described his experience of being deceived online. Catfishing refers to someone who assumes another identity on the internet, often using false photos or information, to interact with others in online settings.

Online grooming: Online grooming occurs when an adult uses electronic communication in a predatory fashion to try to lower a child's inhibitions or heighten their curiosity about sex, with the aim of eventually meeting them in person for the purposes of sexual activity. This can include online chats, sexting, and other forms of communication.

The emotional impact can be as damaging as the deception itself. Around 70% of catfishing victims say they regret sharing personal information, and many say they wish they had been more careful. Whether the goal is attention, revenge, money, or manipulation, catfishers often use photos, names, and even dates of birth stolen from real people.

Online grooming happens when someone builds a relationship with a young person over time, often through messaging apps, games, or social media. Groomers can start on a friendly or supportive note by giving compliments, listening to you, or even sending you gifts, all of which are designed to make you feel special. But it's a trap. Their real goal is to manipulate you, often by asking for personal or explicit photos, pressuring you to meet in person, or threatening you if you don't do what they want. Grooming is a serious crime.

A Save the Children report found that 97% of young adults aged 18–21 in Spain experienced some form of digital sexual violence, such as grooming, sextortion, or the nonconsensual sharing of intimate content when they were minors. Similar to catfishing, more than 80% of grooming cases happen on social media platforms, and 90% take place through private messaging apps like WhatsApp, Snapchat, and Facebook Messenger. Grooming is most common among 12–15-year-olds, with around 70% of victims being teens. Nearly 50% of minors have been approached online by someone they didn't know in a grooming context. Yet less than 40% of grooming incidents are ever reported, and about 35% of teens didn't realise they were being groomed because the interaction felt "normal" or harmless. Groomers often use fake profiles, flattery, small gifts, and private chats to build trust, frequently targeting teens active on social media or gaming platforms in the evenings. Only 15% of teens know how to block or report a groomer, showing how widespread the lack of awareness really is.

One of the most horrifying examples happened in the United Kingdom, where Alexander McCartney, a 26-year-old man, posed as a teenage girl online to groom over 70 children. He convinced several to send explicit videos, and in one case, a 12-year-old girl took her own life after being manipulated and humiliated.

Predators prey on those who are most vulnerable

Loneliness and the desire for connection are powerful emotions that can make teens more vulnerable to online predators. Studies show that predators often target teens who express feelings of isolation or a need for emotional support. For instance, research indicates that children who have experienced neglect are 3.5 times more likely to engage in risky online behaviour, which in turn is associated with a 2.7 times higher risk of online invasive exploitation. Additionally, approximately 85% of online groomers use tactics like flattery and gifts to manipulate minors, exploiting their need for attention and affection. Alarmingly, 80% of children who have been groomed online reported that they felt they could not tell anyone about their experience, citing fear and shame.

Teens who've experienced neglect or trauma are more vulnerable to catfishing and grooming than others. They may be looking for love, attention, or someone to listen, and predators know that. In fact, neglected teens are 3.5 times more likely to fall for online grooming. About 35% of victims report serious emotional damage after being groomed, including anxiety, depression, and suicidal thoughts.

Australian authorities have reported a rise in "sadistic sextortion", where offenders coerce children into producing violent content, sometimes leading to extreme outcomes like self-harm or suicide. These online networks of offenders, being dubbed "crimefluencers", are made up mostly of boys and young men aged 17–20 from English-speaking countries and are not motivated by money or sexual gratification but by sadistic amusement and online status. They target vulnerable pre-teen and teenage girls on social platforms and gaming/chat apps, drawing them into online communities where they are encouraged, coerced, and exploited for violent, degrading, and harmful content. In some reported interactions, victims are pushed to harm themselves, their siblings, others, or even pets, and offenders share or trade this material much like "levels" in an online game to gain popularity within their group. The group of alleged offenders are made up of domestic and international networks, and they use emojis to codify. The alleged offenders operate in both local and international networks, using coded emojis to hide their instructions so parents and adults don't understand the messages.

Did you know? While catfishers target those who are lonely, about 41% of catfishers cite loneliness as a reason for their deceptive online behaviour.

Victims are not who you think, and the outcomes are traumatising

Online grooming has become so common that police in the United Kingdom now record thousands of cases every year, with numbers nearly doubling since 2018. What makes this especially worrying is that victims are often contacted through everyday apps like Snapchat, Instagram, WhatsApp, and gaming platforms, where predators create fake profiles to seem friendly, funny, or supportive. Some offenders talk to dozens of young people at once, slowly building trust through private messages before crossing boundaries. In many cases, the grooming happens quietly over weeks or months, making it hard to notice even for adults. Police and child-safety experts warn that this crime is often hidden in encrypted chats, meaning many teens never realise they're being targeted until the situation feels confusing, uncomfortable, or frightening. These cases show that grooming isn't rare, dramatic, or obvious, as it often looks like "just chatting" at first, which is why so many teens easily fall for it.

While many envision online groomers as adult males, studies reveal a more complex picture. A meta-analysis found that 44% of online sex crime offenders were under 18, and 68% were known to their victims, indicating that peers or acquaintances can also be perpetrators. However, adult males remain predominant in many cases. For instance, research indicates that victims groomed online were mostly girls aged 14–15, with perpetrators being male and up to 25 years older.

The psychological effects on victims can be profound. Approximately 45% of those groomed online report experiencing anxiety or depression. Many victims feel unable to seek help due to fear or shame, with 80% reporting that they couldn't tell anyone about their experience.

In November 2022, a tragic case in Riverside, California, showed the dangers of online deception. Austin Lee Edwards, a 28-year-old former Virginia law enforcement officer, posed online as a 17-year-old to befriend a 15-year-old girl. After establishing a relationship, he travelled across the country to her home, where he murdered her mother and grandparents, set the house on fire, and abducted the teen. Edwards was later killed in a shootout with police. This incident highlights the severe risks associated with online interactions and the importance of staying safe when communicating online.

The predatory behaviours behind catfishing and grooming

The reasons Liz was able to be targeted and manipulated online are complex. Liz thought her friend on Roblox was someone she could trust. They had told her personal things that only another teenage girl would think or feel. She had never experienced someone who understood and got how she thought and felt.

The way these predators gain your trust and then use it against you is terrifying. They exploit your emotions and thinking through deliberate psychological tactics designed to confuse, isolate, and control. The psychology behind online grooming and catfishing involves calculated deception and emotional manipulation. Just like what happened with Liz, offenders use false identities, fabricated stories, and flattery to build a sense of closeness, only to exploit it later. Their motivations vary; some seek control, validation, or attention, while others act out deeper emotional or psychological issues. Whatever the reason, their methods are intentional and predatory, preying on vulnerability and trust to achieve their goals.

Focused on manipulation and control

Both groomers and catfishers use manipulation to control you, but in different ways. Groomers intentionally build emotional connections, using flattery, attention, and gifts to make you feel special and trusted. This creates a dependency that lowers your defences, making it easier for them to control you over time. This process involves deceptive affiliation, where trust is based on lies and false promises. They use fake identities and online impression management, carefully managing their online persona and shaping how others see them to gain trust. By maintaining these lies, they manipulate your feelings or actions and often show addictive signs to the power they hold as they get euphoria or a "high" from seeing their deception succeed.

Rethinking your social contracts: In real life, most of us start by trusting people through an unspoken social contract until they give us a reason not to. But online, it needs to be the other way around. Instead of assuming someone is trustworthy from the start, only trust them once you've confirmed they're legit.

Targeting those who are vulnerable

Grooming is a calculated, predatory process. Groomers are usually those who feel lonely, insecure, or lack strong support systems. They exploit your vulnerabilities to gain trust and eventually abuse or exploit you. This is often easier because of the online disinhibition effect, where people feel freer to lie and manipulate behind the screen, and those they target place greater trust in them because they lack offline cues, such as facial signs, that would indicate deceit. Similarly, some catfishers create fake personas to cope with loneliness or social isolation themselves, while others exploit others' vulnerabilities for personal gain, like revenge or manipulation.

Taking pleasure in the power of being cruel

Groomers often gain a sense of power and domination by controlling your emotions and actions. This control can sometimes bring sadistic pleasure where they have a cruel enjoyment of causing harm or fear. Catfishers may similarly enjoy the power to influence or confuse others, often finding it addictive. Some individuals involved in grooming or catfishing may display traits associated with psychopathy or narcissistic personality disorder, which can include a lack of empathy and a strong desire to manipulate others for personal benefit, causing them to manipulate without remorse. Others may be driven by revenge, jealousy, or anger, using catfishing to harm or humiliate their targets. Both groups exploit the trust they build to meet their own psychological needs or desires.

Living out fantasies online through deception and lies

Deception is central to both grooming and catfishing. Groomers hide their true motives by acting as friends or mentors, keeping their abuse secret from families and authorities, sometimes for months or years. Catfishers use fake identities, sometimes adopting multiple personas in what could be seen as dissociative identity traits to separate their true self from their online lies. For some catfishers, this is also a way to explore or experiment with their gender or sexual identity in a seemingly safer space, even though it involves misleading others. The habitual lying involved may sometimes resemble pathological lying, where the stories become elaborate and compulsive. Being proven that their lies are believable is validation that they are good at what they do.

Most catfishers use the same lie: I or someone close to me is sick, hurt, or in jail.

Exploitation of being free of offline social norms

Both groomers and catfishers take advantage of the anonymity and easy access that online platforms provide. They use popular social media, messaging apps, and games, which are places where teens feel safe and private, to reach and manipulate victims without being easily caught. Social norms and taboos around discussing sexual abuse or deception often let these predators operate in secret. In many ways, this is a form of social engineering, where the abuser tricks victims into trusting them or giving up personal information, much like a hacker tricks people into revealing passwords.

Liz never imagined she could be at risk. She thought she would recognise a predator straight away, that it would be obvious if someone were trying to groom her. But what happened to Liz shows how easy it can be to be deceived when someone online feels so real. Predators know exactly what to say. They build trust slowly, making you feel special, understood, and connected until you start to doubt your own instincts. Even when little things don't add up, they find ways to explain them away. Understanding how this happens is important, but what matters even more is knowing how to protect yourself before it begins.

Check-in: Catfishing and online grooming happen so subtly that it's extremely hard to notice. Consider the signs below and whether you may be experiencing them:

- ❒ Someone I met online avoids video calls, voice notes, and in-person meetings.
- ❒ Their photos look too perfect, repeated, or don't match over time.
- ❒ They say things like "You're the only one who understands me" very early.

- ❒ They quickly push conversations into private chats or disappearing messages.
- ❒ They ask me to keep our conversations secret from friends, parents, caregivers, or teachers.
- ❒ They get jealous, controlling, or upset when I talk to others or when I don't reply quickly.
- ❒ They ask personal questions about my family, school, location, or daily routine.
- ❒ They test boundaries with flirting, sexual jokes, comments, or requests that make me uneasy or unsure.
- ❒ They pressure me to share photos, videos, or personal information.
- ❒ I feel confused, anxious, guilty, or uncomfortable after talking to them.

Consider the number you can say that you are experiencing:

0–2 ticks: Low risk and probably safe, but still trust your instincts and keep boundaries strong.
3–5 ticks: High risk, and something isn't right. Slow things down, stop sharing personal info, and talk to a trusted adult.
6+ ticks: Very high risk, and this is likely to be catfishing or grooming. Stop engaging, block the person, save evidence, and get help immediately.

How technology is used as a weapon to catfish and groom you

Liz was online just to have fun and enjoy talking to friends. She felt like these friends understood her and were people she could trust. Liz never thought she could be so easily targeted online. As outlined earlier, "crimefluencers" and online crime gangsters are on the rise. These cyber criminals hunt young children, especially young girls, for sadistic exploitation or to get them to commit acts of violence against themselves or against others. "Crimefluencers" and sometimes just people online will use catfishing and online grooming techniques and strategies to recruit their victims. They research the best approaches and learn how to use technology to manipulate you as easily as possible. There are several steps you can take to avoid falling victim to catfishing and online grooming.

Recognising fake profiles

Cyber criminals who engage in catfishing and online grooming don't use their true identities online. They often hide behind fake accounts to hunt their victims using those social engineering tactics in which they leverage building trust with their victims. For this reason, it is important to learn how to spot fake and suspicious accounts. Common signs of fake and suspicious accounts are that the face in the profile photo is too charismatic (male) or too model-like (female), or the bio about the person's life is too good to be true. Unlike real accounts, where there is a history of posting and commenting, fake and suspicious accounts are typically new and contain fewer photos and posts, which are often recycled across social media platforms.

Fake or suspicious accounts often contain inconsistent details in the profile, i.e., hobbies, job, age, or location, that don't add up, especially when details shared in one profile don't align with the details shared on another profile. Those who operate fake or suspicious accounts tend to progress in relationships very quickly by expressing raw emotions that normally take time to develop naturally, so saying things like "I love you" and "you are special to me" after exchanging just a few messages makes no sense. Also, they always have an excuse ready if you try to call them on the phone or video chat with them, to keep the communication under their control.

To verify the authenticity of these profiles, you can use reverse image search. You should also check the photo metadata for missing or odd data, and the GPS data for consistency with the information on the profile. Aside from investigating the profile photo's originality, you should also analyse the account's social media activity. Go through some of their social media posts and find out if they are consistent in their comments on others' posts and their use of tags and likes.

Managing online friendships safely

Falling victim to catfishing and online grooming starts with accepting a friendship request, so be extra vigilant when accepting requests from strangers. Before accepting their friendship requests, verify their identities. Ask them: from where do they know you, i.e., school, sport, or swimming lessons? Ask them also: who are the mutual friends they share? If you end up accepting their invitations, don't trust them with your private information, like your photos, or personally identifying information, like your home address, school, or the places you frequent. Be proactive in managing your privacy settings. Make your social media accounts private, and limit who can message you or follow you. If you have been tagged in a photo or a post, review those photos and posts and dissociate from those photos and posts if you don't approve of them.

Read more information on privacy settings in Chapter 2: Smartphone Privacy, Security Settings, and Your Identifying Information.

Read more information on recognising fake profiles online in Chapter 4: Becoming Resilient to Cyberbullying and Trolling.

Setting boundaries in your communication with others is an important step in protecting yourself from falling victim to catfishing and online grooming crimes. It is okay to say no. You don't owe anyone a thing. Say no to an unknown contact who asks you to download a file, and never share your password or verification codes with anyone, including your best friends. If someone is a bit pushy, that is a red flag. Why are they keen on you? Most, if not all, social media platforms allow users to block other users, mute them, ignore them, restrict their access to you, and/or report them. Use those features and in-app functions to ensure you enjoy a safe social media experience.

Identifying and addressing uncomfortable online interactions

Catfishers and online groomers try to recruit you by making you feel special or unique. They know you crave attention and respond positively to compliments, so they give you lots of attention and flattery. They also try to discourage you from talking to your family and friends about them, isolating you from your close ties. They may also make the conversation with them very personal or inappropriate, testing your boundaries along the way to see which will work and which won't work. If you try to slow things down, they may try to guilt you into doing what they want by saying things like "don't you trust me?" or "if you love me, you would do this". To protect yourself from manipulation by catfishers and online groomers, use the blocking, muting, ignoring, restricting, and reporting features and in-app functions to stop interactions that make you feel uncomfortable. If you plan to report a connection, take screenshots of the interaction or save the messages, as this evidence will likely be required during any investigation. There are websites in most countries that have a robust and effective abuse reporting mechanism, which you can use to report abuse if you have experienced it:

- Australia: eSafety Commissioner website https://www.esafety.gov.au/report
- United States: Internet Crime Complaints Centre website https://www.ic3.gov
- United Kingdom: Safer Internet website https://saferinternet.org.uk/online-issue/reporting

If you are using Roblox, involve your parents or caregivers in your gaming experience. Get them to sign up to use the platform and link their account to yours. They can protect you in several ways using the platform's parental control features. They can control the content to which you are exposed, block an experience, select content type (i.e., mild, moderate, and restricted) based on your age, deny someone the ability to direct text chat with you, or block a connection to remove them from your connections list.

Understanding and respecting consent

Understanding and respecting consent is a fundamental aspect of healthy relationships. Consent is giving permission. It must be clear, mutual, and ongoing. Consent applies to everything you do online, including the sharing of photos, intimate disclosure, and the reposting of others' content. You have the right to refuse to give someone consent (dissent) to share a photo of you that you don't approve of. If you had initially given consent and later discovered you no longer want that photo of you to be shared, you can change your mind about the consent you initially gave. Be alert to being coerced into consenting to sharing something you don't want to share. You should not feel pressured, guilted into, or threatened into giving consent. Being in a healthy online relationship means both parties respect each other's boundaries and feel comfortable saying no to a request without fear, guilt, or intimidation. Violation of these rules means the interaction is not respectful and should end immediately, and perhaps be reported.

How to use image search to catch a catfish

In addition to conducting reverse image searches using TinEye, you can also use Google Reverse Image Search to catch a catfish. [1] Take a screenshot of the profile photo or copy the link to the photo. [2] Go to images.google.com. [3] Click the camera icon and upload the photo or the link to it. [4] If the photo appears under different names or across different websites, or appears in other people's profiles, then it is most likely fake. If the image is AI-generated or appears on a modelling or stock photo site, then it is also likely to be fake.

Read more information on how to search for fake images or information online in Chapter 9: How to Avoid Fake News and Online Misinformation

What to do if you have been catfished or groomed online

Finding out that someone you trusted online wasn't who they claimed to be or realising you've been slowly manipulated can feel shocking, embarrassing, and overwhelming. That's exactly what happened to Liz, who thought she had finally found someone who understood her, only to discover she had been taken advantage of. Like many teens, Liz didn't do anything wrong. The person on the other side of the screen carefully built trust, crossed boundaries bit by bit, and made it hard to speak up. If this has happened to you, you are not alone; it is not your fault, and you can take action to resolve the situation.

1 Stop all contact and don't respond

If you think someone online is catfishing or grooming you, the first step is to cut off all contact completely. Block them on every app, game, or platform where they've messaged you. Don't reply to their messages, even if they say sorry, act sweetly, or try to make you feel guilty.

Groomers and catfishers often try to keep you talking so they can stay in control. The more you engage, the harder it can be to walk away, and the more pressure they may put on you. So don't give them that chance.

Trust your instincts, and if something feels off, it probably is. Ending the conversation and blocking them is the safest move.

> **Legal tip:** It's an offence for an adult to start an online relationship with someone under the age of 16 with the intention of having a sexual relationship with them. It's against the law and a *crime* even if the adult and the child never meet in real life.

2 Protect your accounts, save and record everything

Make your personal details (such as your phone number, date of birth, and email) private in your account settings so strangers can't access them. You can also check whether your email has been leaked in a data breach using websites like https://haveibeenpwned.com/.

If someone has made a fake profile pretending to be you or someone else, don't ignore it. Take screenshots of the profile, usernames, and messages. Save all chats, photos, or posts, even if they're upsetting, because they might be needed as evidence. Record where and when things happened, like which app and what date.

3 Block and report the person

If you've been catfished or groomed, it's important to block the person immediately on all apps, games, or platforms where they've contacted you. Blocking stops communication and helps protect your safety. Most platforms also have tools to report fake profiles, grooming, threats, or inappropriate messages; use them right away.

If the person is trying to build a relationship, especially one that feels intense, romantic, or overly personal, and they are older or pushing for things that don't feel right, it could be illegal grooming. This includes:

- ☑ Saying they love you or want to date you even though you just met online
- ☑ Asking you to keep your chats a secret from adults
- ☑ Trying to meet up in person, especially if they're an adult and you're underage
- ☑ Asking for sexual photos or saying things that are sexual

If someone is doing any of these things, stop talking to them, block them, and tell a trusted adult immediately. It is never your fault. Groomers are manipulative and often pretend to care to get what they want.

If you've shared money or personal content, don't send anything else and contact your bank or payment service for help. If the person is threatening you or you feel unsafe, report it to local police or a national cyber crime agency right away.

Remember

If you are being **blackmailed** and someone is threatening to post pictures, videos, or messages unless you give them more content or money, do not give in. That only encourages them.

- ✓ If you're under 18, tell a trusted adult, teacher, or youth counsellor and report it to a child protection or cyber-safety agency (like CyberTipline in the United States, CEOP in the United Kingdom, or ACCCE in Australia).
- ✓ If you're 18 or older, report the person on the platform and seek help from an online safety agency or legal support service in your country.

Legal tip: Even without threats, sharing your private images without your consent is illegal in many places. Report it to the platform and contact an image-based abuse service or online safety agency, as they may be able to help you remove the content.

4 Reach out for support

If you've experienced catfishing or online grooming, it's important to know you're not alone and that there is help available. Talking to someone you trust, like a friend, family member, or school counsellor, can make a big difference. Sometimes just sharing what's happened can ease feelings of loneliness, fear, or embarrassment. Many teens who have been catfished or groomed struggle with trusting others afterwards or feel ashamed, but remember it's never your fault. Online groomers and catfishers are expert manipulators and target those who are most trusting and haven't experienced it before.

Online grooming and catfishing can have serious effects on your mental health. Some victims feel angry, scared, or worried that private images or messages might be shared without their permission. It's normal to feel overwhelmed, but reaching out for support can help you heal and stay safe.

Because groomers and catfishers often rely on secrecy and shame to control you, they want you to stay silent. If you're feeling uncomfortable or unsafe in an online friendship or relationship, tell a trusted adult, even if it's hard. They want to help you, and sharing is the first step to stopping the abuse.

Different countries have support services and hotlines for young people experiencing online abuse, grooming, or exploitation. Look up your local resources to report what's happening and get professional help. If you ever feel in immediate danger, contact your local emergency services.

Also, think about your offline safety. Sometimes online harassment or stalking can turn into real-world threats. Be careful about who knows your location or daily routines and take steps to protect your privacy in both online and offline spaces.

Search online for "[Your country] online abuse hotline"; "[Your country] cyberbullying support"; "[Your country] report online grooming"

Conclusion

Groomers and catfishers use fake identities to deceive individuals online. This chapter offered guidance on how to recognise catfishing attempts, verify online identities, and avoid being manipulated into dangerous situations. It also detailed online grooming tactics and how predators build trust and isolate victims to manipulate them. The chapter also equipped teens with the knowledge and skills to detect and prevent exploitation by helping them recognise fake profiles, manage online friendships safely, identify and address uncomfortable online interactions, and understand and respect consent. Remember, trusting your instincts is key. If something feels off or too good to be true, it probably is. Take your time, stay connected with people you trust, and don't be afraid to block or report anyone who makes you feel uncomfortable.

Key terms

- Catfishing
- Online grooming
- Sadistic sextortion
- Crimefluencers
- Social contract
- Narcissistic
- Anonymity
- Social engineering
- Cyber criminals
- Fake accounts
- Online consent
- Reverse image search

Bibliography

Abcarian, R. (2022, December 7). *Catfishing, sextortion and a Riverside tragedy*. Los Angeles Times. https://www.latimes.com/opinion/story/2022-12-07/catfishing-riverside-sextortion-killings

Alund, N.N. (2022, November 29). *What is catfishing? Why do people catfish? Here's what you need to know*. USA Today. https://www.usatoday.com/story/news/nation/2022/11/29/what-is-catfishing-why-do-people-catfish/10794619002/

Australian Broadcasting Corporation. (2024, October 26). *Alexander McCartney sentenced to life in prison for manslaughter after blackmailing thousands of girls*. ABC News. https://www.abc.net.au/news/2024-10-26/alexander-mccartney-sentenced-to-life-in-prison-for-manslaughter/104521346

Australian Centre to Counter Child Exploitation. (2020). *Online child sexual exploitation: Understanding community awareness, perceptions, attitudes and preventative behaviours research report*. https://www.accce.gov.au/sites/default/files/2021-02/ACCCE_Research-Report_OCE.pdf

Australian Competition and Consumer Commission. (2026, February 26). *Understand how criminals exploit online relationships and inflict heartache*. https://www.accc.gov.au/media-release/understand-how-criminals-exploit-online-relationships-and-inflict-heartache

Australian Federal Police. (2024, September 6). *AFP warning over rise of sadistic sextortion online*. https://www.afp.gov.au/news-centre/media-release/afp-warning-over-rise-sadistic-sextortion-online

Ballard, J. (2025, May 12). *10 startling catfishing statistics: What you need to know*. DatingNews. https://www.datingnews.com/industry-trends/catfishing-statistics

Bravehearts. (n.d.). *Online child exploitation*. https://bravehearts.org.au/about-child-sexual-abuse/online-child-expoitation/

Bravehearts. (n.d.). *Online risks: Child exploitation and grooming statistics and facts*. https://bravehearts.org.au/research-lobbying/stats-facts/online-risks-child-exploitation-grooming/

Department of Education and Training Victoria. (n.d.). *A school guide to understanding grooming*. https://www.education.vic.gov.au/Documents/about/programs/bullystoppers/smgrooming.pdf

Deutsche Welle. (2024, October 25). *Life sentence for UK's biggest online catfishing predator*. https://www.dw.com/en/online-predator-gets-life-in-uks-biggest-catfishing-case/a-70602985

Du Toit, M. (2024, February 13). *Catfishing statistics*. Review42. https://review42.com/resources/catfishing-statistics/

Emery, C.R., Wong, P.W.C., Haden-Pawlowski, V., Pui, C., Wong, G., Kwok, S., Liu, A.Y., & Abdullah, A. (2023). Neglect, online invasive exploitation, and childhood sexual abuse in Hong Kong: Breaking the links. *Child Abuse & Neglect, 144*, 106591. https://doi.org/10.1016/j.chiabu.2023.106591

Fontaine, G. (2026, February 13). *Online grooming statistics*. https://gitnux.org/online-grooming-statistics

Gan, X., Qin, K.N., Xiang, G.X., & Jin, X. (2023). The relationship between parental neglect and cyberbullying perpetration among Chinese adolescent: The sequential role of cyberbullying victimization and internet gaming disorder. *Frontiers in Public Health, 11*, 1128123. https://doi.org/10.3389/fpubh.2023.1128123

Haidt, J. (2024, November 1). *Nearly two children a day groomed by online predators in the UK*. The Times. https://www.thetimes.co.uk/article/almost-two-children-a-day-groomed-by-online-predators-6rv83hvbl

Jonsson, L.S., Fredlund, C., Priebe, G., Wadsby, M., & Svedin, C.G. (2019). Online sexual abuse of adolescents by a perpetrator met online: A cross-sectional study. *Child and Adolescent Psychiatry and Mental Health, 13*, 32. https://doi.org/10.1186/s13034-019-0292-1

Kids Helpline. (2019, February 15). *Understanding online grooming.* https://kidshelpline.com.au/parents/issues/understanding-online-grooming

Malwarebytes. (n.d.). *What is catfishing online: Signs & how to protect yourself.* https://www.malwarebytes.com/cybersecurity/basics/catfishing

McMahon, L., Singleton, T., & Hayes, G. (2024, November 28). *"It's so easy to lie": A fifth of children use fake age on social media.* BBC News. https://www.bbc.com/news/articles/cn4v52ezx17o

Meredith, R. (2024, November 16). *UK's largest catfishing case involving child exploitation.* BBC News. https://www.bbc.com/news/articles/cly2z89ep71o

O'Carroll, L. (2024, October 25). *Northern Ireland man jailed for life after abusing children online.* The Guardian. https://www.theguardian.com/uk-news/2024/oct/25/alexander-mccartney-northern-ireland-man-jailed-for-life-abusing-children-online

Olbrycht-Palmer, J. (2024, October 29). *Crimefluencers hunting young girls for sadistic online exploitation, AFP chief warns.* News.com.au. https://www.news.com.au/national/crime/crimefluencers-hunting-young-girls-for-sadistic-online-exploitation-afp-chief-warns/news-story/62fa772c3c059cb08240f1ae3b34b602

Our Rescue. (2025, December 5). *The psychology behind online predators.* https://ourrescue.org/resources/child-exploitation/online-exploitation/the-psychology-behind-online-predators

Patchin, J.W. (2013, February 7). *Catfishing as a form of cyberbullying.* Cyberbullying Research Center. https://cyberbullying.org/catfishing-as-a-form-of-cyberbullying

Pew Research Center. (2025, December 15). *Teens and Cyberbullying 2022.* https://www.pewresearch.org/internet/2022/12/15/teens-and-cyberbullying-2022/

Proofpoint. (n.d.). *Catfishing.* https://www.proofpoint.com/au/threat-reference/catfishing

Raffo, F. (2025, July 7). *97% of young people report having suffered some type of sexual violence in digital environments when they were minors.* El País. https://elpais.com/sociedad/2025-07-07/el-97-de-jovenes-afirma-haber-sufrido-algun-tipo-de-violencia-sexual-en-entornos-digitales-cuando-eran-menores.html

Rahman-Jones, I. (2024, November 1). *"Snapchat most-used app for grooming," says NSPCC.* BBC News. https://www.bbc.com/news/articles/cze3p1j710ko

Save the Children. (2025, July 9). *One in 5 young people in Spain report being victims of AI deepfakes with almost all reporting sexual violence online.* https://www.savethechildren.net/news/one-5-young-people-spain-report-being-victims-ai-deepfakes-almost-all-reporting-sexual

Schmidt, F., Varese, F., & Bucci, S. (2023). Understanding the prolonged impact of online sexual abuse occurring in childhood. *Frontiers in Psychology, 14*, 1281996. https://doi.org/10.3389/fpsyg.2023.1281996

Sutton, S., & Finkelhor, D. (2024). Perpetrators' identity in online crimes against children: A meta-analysis. *Trauma, Violence & Abuse, 25*(3), 1756–1768. https://doi.org/10.1177/15248380231194072

Sydney Times. (2025, October 30). *New crime influencers threat: AFP Commissioner Krissy Barrett warns of online sadism targeting youth.* https://citynews.com.au/2025/foreign-actors-cohesion-priority-for-nations-top-cop/

Tan, M. (2026, February 16). *Online grooming statistics.* WorldMetrics. https://worldmetrics.org/online-grooming-statistics

Thorn. (2025). *Commodified sexual interactions involving minors: New data on evolving dynamics in technology-facilitated child sexual exploitation.* https://info.thorn.org/hubfs/Research/Thorn_CommodifiedSexualInteractionsInvolvingMinors_Apr2025.pdf

Thorn. (n.d.). *Grooming and sextortion.* https://www.thorn.org/research/grooming-and-sextortion/

Touma, R. (2024, September 7). *AFP warns of rising cases of sadistic child sextortion.* The Guardian. https://www.theguardian.com/technology/article/2024/sep/07/australia-federal-police-sadistic-child-sextortion-warning

Tuohy, W. (2021, June 7). *Jump in sexual assaults of children groomed online.* RCH News. https://blogs.rch.org.au/news/jump-in-sexual-assaults-of-children-groomed-online/

Turnbull, T. (2025, October 19). *Australian girls being 'hunted' by online crime gangs to commit violent acts.* BBC News. https://www.bbc.com/news/articles/c0qpl7v7p0jo

UNSW Sydney. (2024, May 7). *More than 300 million child victims of online sexual abuse globally: Report.* https://www.unsw.edu.au/newsroom/news/2024/05/more-than-300-million-child-victims-of-online-sexual-abuse-globally-report

Wefers, S., Dieseth, T., George, E., Øverland, I., Jolapara, J., McAree, C., & Findlater, D. (2024). Understanding and deterring online child grooming: A qualitative study. *Sexual Offending (Trier, Germany), 19*, e13147. https://doi.org/10.5964/sotrap.13147

8 How to recognise and respond to hate speech and radicalised views

"Eat your food, bruh," Tso called out, as he got up from his seat, lifted his tray, and walked to sit at the table in front of him, where Daw, an African-looking boy, was sitting alone, feeling lonely and visibly upset in the overcrowded, chaotic, and loud juvenile correctional centre's canteen. "If you don't start eating your food, it will be gone in no time," Tso continued. "Look, they are already eyeing it," Tso said. "I am not hungry," Daw said. "Up to you, but the next meal is at 8 am," Tso explained. Seeing Daw touch his food, Tso asked, "How did you end up here?" "The cops accused me of plotting to kill our neighbour," Daw answered. "What, that is insane!" Tso responded in shock, "Tell me what happened." "I don't want to talk about it," 14-year-old Daw replied.

***

The following week, after Daw's parents and two of his siblings visited him in juvi, he told Tso his story as they walked back to their cell, having finished school for the day. Daw's story began when his family's next-door neighbour brought the police to his family's home, accusing him of stealing his car. The neighbour said he first saw him the day before, hanging out with his African friends at KFC after school, and again later that day with the same group outside his house. Daw denied any involvement in the theft of the neighbour's car and argued he had never done anything wrong. Daw was not taken into custody because the police officer at the time received word that the youths who stole the car were arrested while trying to torch it, but the encounter with the police left him consumed by his own sense of victimhood.

***

Trying to make sense of this, Daw searched for information about racism on social media. As he deep-dived into the topic, he became engulfed in social media content that made him angrier each day, yet connected. The people he followed on Telegram were sympathetic to his personal grievance against his neighbour and the police, and their speeches not only made sense but made him feel he belonged. Spending hours daily

DOI: 10.4324/9781003681731-9

watching these people's videos, he became convinced he should correct the injustice inflicted upon him. Feeding on months of hateful content that brainwashed him into thinking wrongdoing is justified in his case, he reached a 'tipping point' where he searched how to assemble a gun (DIY) from available materials. It was this search that led to his arrest and to the police charge of plotting to murder. The subsequent piecing together of evidence resulted in his conviction.

You are constantly targeted online

Recent global studies show a concerning trend where hate speech and extremist content are no longer rare online; they're part of what many young people see every day. According to a global survey, 54% of teens said they had faced online risks like hate speech, cyberbullying, or violent threats, and 38% had seen extremist or violent content in just one year.

Another study found that more than half (53%) of all teens had come across hate speech. One in three teens had seen images or videos promoting terrorism. For some groups, the risks are even greater. For example, 31% of LGBTQ+ teens reported being directly targeted by hate speech, and 80% had seen harmful or hateful content in a 12-month period.

What is hate speech and radicalisation?

Hate speech: Online hate refers to any derogatory or hostile messages directed at an individual or group based on characteristics that are not changeable, such as race, religion, ethnicity, gender, sexual orientation, or disability.

Radicalisation: Online radicalisation refers to the process by which individuals develop stronger support for extremist ideologies or behaviours through online interactions and exposure to related content. This may include adopting extremist viewpoints, participating in online extremist communities, and, in some cases, being incited to engage in acts of violence.

Real-life cases show how serious this problem can become. In Australia, the police have indicated that the Bondi terrorist attacker, Naveed Akram, may have been influenced by online extreme rhetoric connected to a religious hate preacher. In France, a 12-year-old boy started watching religious videos, but within weeks, he had found his way into encrypted chat groups full of violent propaganda, including bomb-making instructions and graphic images. Experts say this kind of content can warp a young person's values and can even steer them towards violent extremist ideologies.

Extremist messages don't always look like hate right away

Sometimes, extremist messages are hidden inside other toxic beliefs. A report from the United Kingdom found that almost half of young men aged 16–24 had a positive view of influencer Andrew Tate, whose content often promotes misogyny and authoritarian thinking. Experts warn that these ideas can be a gateway into more extreme worldviews.

Youth radicalisation is now growing fast across many countries. In France, minors made up 20% of terrorism prosecutions in 2024, a significant increase from the previous two years. In Belgium, 18% of extremist threats involved young people. In the United Kingdom, 82 teens under 18 were arrested for terrorism-related charges in just one year, compared to only 12 in 2019. Australia has seen similar patterns, with 20% of its top counter-terrorism cases involving teens, including 35 minors investigated since 2020.

Teens are the most at-risk group for hate speech and radicalisation

Around the world, teens are spending more time online than ever. In the United States, 96% of 13–17-year-olds go online daily, and nearly half are online almost constantly. That constant exposure increases the likelihood of encountering harmful content, especially when algorithms on platforms like YouTube, TikTok, and Discord recommend more extreme material over time.

Online hate speech is becoming part of everyday life for many young people, even though most adults don't see just how common it is. A UK study found that 1 in 5 kids aged 9–16 years had seen hateful content online, things like racist, sexist, or anti-LGBTQ+ messages. It might be in a meme, a comment, or a video that seems funny at first, but beneath the surface, it spreads messages that hurt people and divide communities.

Meanwhile, real-world examples show that hate online doesn't always stay online. In Australia, every single counter-terrorism case has involved a teen or young adult, including 37 individuals under 17, with the youngest just 12 years old. The tragic Bondi terrorist attack, which is one of the most confronting acts of violence in recent Australian history, cost 15 Australians their lives, and is no exception. Many of those involved in terrorism-related activities were exposed to extremist content through platforms like TikTok, Discord, and Telegram. Teens are especially vulnerable to radical ideas because their brains are still developing. It's normal to feel emotional or impulsive, but that also makes it easier for harmful messages to take hold, especially when online spaces, algorithms, and echo chambers keep repeating the same extreme ideas. What starts as casual scrolling can turn into deep involvement in extremist groups without you even realising it.

One especially concerning case involved a 15-year-old girl who became radicalised in just a few short weeks. She was spending a lot of time online, where she found extremist content that seemed powerful or exciting at first, but was actually full of hate. Before anyone noticed, she started to believe the ideas and even planned to travel overseas to join a violent group. This wasn't a video game or a fantasy; it was real, and it nearly cost her everything.

Alarms have been raised about teens using AI tools to find instructions on making weapons or pledging loyalty to extremist causes. It's a reminder that what we see and who we talk to online matters, and even a few clicks in the wrong direction can have dangerous consequences.

In another case, a 17-year-old boy used AI tools, such as advanced chatbots, to look up how to make weapons and get ammunition. He wasn't just curious. He had already been spending time in online spaces where extreme beliefs were shared and encouraged. These echo chambers made him feel like he belonged, but they were also normalising hate and violence. The concerning part is that it all started online, in seemingly normal chat apps, game servers, or social media platforms.

Did you know? Online hate has negative effects on the well-being of both *victims* and those who *observe* it happening, including "depression, isolation, paranoia, social anxiety, self-doubt, disappointment, loneliness, and lack of confidence".

Where you feel safest is where extremists target you

It might not seem obvious, but the way online platforms work can actually push people towards more extreme content. Apps like YouTube, TikTok, Instagram, and Facebook use algorithms to recommend videos and posts you might like based on what you've watched before. But sometimes, these systems lead people down a certain path without them even noticing. What starts as a harmless video can slowly turn into content that's more hateful, conspiratorial, or violent. This is called algorithmic radicalisation, and it's one of the ways extremist ideas can quietly sneak into your feed.

Gaming platforms can also be a hotspot for recruitment. Extremist groups have been known to use in-game chats, livestreams, and private servers to connect with young players and slowly gain their trust. They might act friendly at first, but their goal is to pull teens into other platforms, like Discord, where they can share far-right propaganda and even glorify things like school shootings or terrorism. In the United Kingdom, police and intelligence agencies have raised alarms about this tactic, especially during school holidays, when teens are more online and support networks are weaker. Instead of openly preaching hateful messages, extremists often build relationships first, using code words, memes, and subtle symbols to get around platform rules.

This isn't just a problem in one country; it's happening worldwide. In Australia, nearly all counter-terrorism cases investigated since 2020 have involved teens or young adults, with more than 35 individuals aged 12–17. It's been reported that 13% of UK terrorism cases now involve under-18s, triple what they were just three years ago. In Singapore, the time it takes for someone to become self-radicalised has dropped by half from 24 months before 2015 to just 12 months today, thanks to fast-moving online content. Many have been radicalised online, especially those struggling with loneliness, trauma, neurodiversity, or mental health issues. Recruiters often exploit people's need for connection, slowly introducing harmful ideas in places like Roblox, TikTok, Instagram, and Telegram.

The psychological mind tricks behind hate speech and radicalisation

Daw started out just watching videos and stories about racism. But that innocent scrolling quickly spiralled into something bigger because social media learns what you look at and then keeps pushing more of it your way. That's how hate speech makes you think it's normal to act that way and how you start doing and saying things you would never have done before. It's a psychological game designed to target you.

The people doing this online know exactly how to play with your emotions and what gets young people like Daw hooked on reading more content. They tap into your grievances and slowly make extreme ideas feel normal. Radicalisation rarely occurs in a single dramatic moment. It usually starts quietly, pulling you in step by step through subtle tricks that twist your thinking without you noticing. And the people behind it aren't always angry or obvious. Sometimes they come across as funny, supportive, or even inspirational. But behind the screen, they're working to shape how you think, feel, and act, especially during your teenage years, when you're still figuring out who you are.

Black-and-white thinking and why extremists want you to pick a side

People who spread hate or extremist ideas often see the world in extreme, black-and-white terms like "us versus them" or "good versus evil". They believe their group, whether it's based on race, religion, politics, or gender, is superior and that everyone else is a threat. This way of thinking fuels their need to blame, divide, and dehumanise others.

Why do they do this? Because it's psychologically easier. Life is messy and complicated, but hate groups offer simple answers that make the world feel more understandable. Instead of dealing with uncertainty or injustice thoughtfully, they cling to rigid beliefs that give them a sense of control, purpose, and identity.

To get you hooked, they use emotionally explosive content like shocking headlines, made-up stories, or graphic images meant to spark fear, anger, or disgust, especially against groups like refugees, religious minorities, women, or the LGBTQ+ community. The goal is to trigger your emotions so strongly that you don't stop to question the message. When you're upset, it's harder to think logically.

Extremists love creating emotional extremes. They will tell you things like: "We're the good guys", or "They're the enemy".

They turn complicated problems like poverty, war, or inequality into something that sounds easy to solve by blaming a single group. These ideas can feel powerful, especially when you're already feeling frustrated, lost, or angry.

The power game is all about controlling you

Some of the people who spread hate or radical ideas online aren't just trying to share opinions; they're trying to control others. For them, gaining followers or manipulating teens isn't about belief; it's about power, influence, and sometimes even fame. The more people they recruit, the more important they feel.

The internet gives these people the perfect hiding spot. Behind a screen, they can act like mentors, leaders, or even friends without having to face any real-world consequences. They often target you at your most vulnerable moments, because they know it's easier to influence someone who's struggling with loneliness, rejection, anxiety, or confusion.

Their methods are slow, sneaky, and psychological. Just like grooming or cult recruitment, they start by building trust. Maybe they seem supportive, cool, or understanding at first. Over time, they introduce more extreme ideas to slowly influence how you see the world, other people, and even yourself. It doesn't feel like brainwashing, but that's exactly what's happening.

> **Extremists will take serious issues like poverty, job loss, or mental health and twist them into simple, toxic messages**: "Things were fine until they showed up", or "People like them are the reason you're suffering".

One of their favourite tricks is blaming others for complex problems. These lies feel emotionally satisfying because they offer someone to blame. But they're misleading and dangerous. They distract you from the real issues and push you towards hate instead of understanding.

How they lure you with friendship and belonging

Hate groups and radical influencers usually don't start by yelling offensive opinions. In fact, they often begin by acting funny, chill, or even supportive. They share memes, inside jokes, or relatable posts that make them seem harmless or even cool. If you're feeling alone or misunderstood, it's easy to feel like you've found someone who gets you. That's exactly what they want.

> **For further information on online grooming, which involves individuals who adopt false identities to build relationships and influence others towards certain behaviours or beliefs**: Chapter 7: Recognising and Responding to Catfishing and Online Grooming

Once they've earned your trust, they start slipping in darker ideas by slowly introducing hate, blame, or conspiracy theories. It might not feel like a big deal at first because it's framed as a joke, an "edgy" opinion, or a bold truth. But before you realise it, you're being nudged towards dangerous beliefs. What started as a meme becomes manipulative. Why does this work so well? Because everyone, especially teens, wants to belong.

Extremists make you feel like you are part of something important, something special, using messages like: "We're not like everyone else", "You're finally seeing the truth", or "The others are just sheep".

This taps into a psychological concept called social identity theory, where being part of a group shapes how you see yourself and others. When you feel accepted by a group, you're more likely to adopt their ideas, even if those ideas are harmful.

These tactics feel empowering. You think you're becoming stronger, smarter, and more independent. But, in reality, you're being manipulated into spreading hate, often without even noticing it.

When they make their issues your problem

A lot of the people spreading hate online aren't as tough as they seem. In fact, many of them are carrying around deep feelings of failure, rejection, or trauma. Instead of dealing with those feelings in healthy ways, they project their pain onto others, blaming people from different races, religions, or communities for everything that's gone wrong in their lives.

For them, hate becomes a kind of emotional escape. It gives them someone to blame and a false sense of control. That's why these individuals often hang out in online spaces where people feel angry, left out, or ignored.

Extremists will feed you information that contains toxic beliefs, but sounds like answers to society's problems: "You're suffering because of them", or "They're the reason your life is hard".

Feeling misunderstood, excluded, or anxious is completely normal, especially during your teen years. But radicalisers know this, and they take advantage of it. They appear kind at first, like someone who finally understands what you're going through. They offer comfort, validation, and a sense of belonging. But once they've got your trust, they start feeding you their anger, shaping how you think and who you blame until their problems start becoming yours.

You become the "Chosen One"

Some radicalisers act like they've got all the answers. They come across as confident, clever, even heroic, like they're the only ones who really see what's going on. They might call themselves "woke", "awakened", or say everyone else is blind or brainwashed. But behind all that confidence is often narcissism, where they believe that they're superior and deserve followers.

Online, these personalities can grow fast. They gain likes, followers, and praise, and build echo chambers where no one challenges their views. To a teen figuring out who they are, these people might seem exciting or inspirational. They'll tell you that you are special, you have been chosen because of how great you are, or that you are part of something important.

That can feel amazing, especially if you've felt invisible or unsure of your place. It makes you feel validated. But what they're really doing is using your need for identity and purpose to pull you in. They don't want you to think for yourself. They want you to follow them.

Some people online try to convince you that violence or cruelty is not just okay; it's heroic, as you are part of something powerful. They say things like, "We're defending our way of life", or "They deserve it". This is called moral disengagement, which is a psychological trick where people convince themselves that hurting others is justified, even noble.

Radicalisers use this to reframe violence as something brave. They'll share videos of attackers and call them "freedom fighters", "warriors", or "martyrs". Over time, this can rewire how you feel about violence, making it seem meaningful instead of wrong.

How the repetition tricks your brain

Online, repetition is powerful. The more you see or hear something, even if it's false, the more familiar and believable it feels. This is called the illusory truth effect. Radicalisers know this, and they use it to their advantage.

You might start by seeing a motivational quote or a seemingly harmless political meme. But over time, the content slowly shifts from frustration to blame, from edgy jokes to hateful messages, then on to conspiracy theories or even violent calls to action. It's like a drip-feed of dangerous ideas.

The more you're exposed to this content, the more normal it starts to feel. That's called gradual desensitisation: as your brain gets used to extreme messages, the things that once shocked you, no longer do.

And here's the problem: platforms like TikTok, YouTube, and Instagram often recommend similar content, creating an echo chamber where all you see is one perspective. Without realising it, you're being nudged further in a specific direction.

Understanding how Daw, who never thought he'd be at risk of being influenced, was pulled in so quickly shows how easily anyone can be caught off guard. He wasn't looking for extreme content. It found him, mixed in with the everyday videos and posts he thought were harmless. His experience is a reminder that hate and radicalisation aren't always dangerous at first. It looks like you must act to help people.

Hate speech and radicalisation are most dangerous when they sneak in quietly. They can be hidden in jokes, friendly chats, or shared feelings of anger. Once they take hold, they can change how you see other people, how you treat them, and even how you see yourself. That's why it's so important to spot these sneaky signs early. When you do, you can question harmful messages, stand up for yourself, and protect your friends.

People who spread hate don't just share ideas; they work to change how you think, feel, and view the world. They do it slowly, using psychology to earn your trust, twist your values, and turn you against others. By the time you realise what's happening, you might already feel loyal, attached, or stuck, and that's what makes it so hard to break free.

Check-in: Are you experiencing indicators of potentially becoming a victim of participating in hate speech and radicalisation?

- ❒ Are you seeing the same messages or themes repeatedly?
- ❒ Is your feed showing only one type of opinion?
- ❒ Do someone's online posts and messages always blame one group for everything?
- ❒ Does someone online act like they're always right and everyone else is wrong?
- ❒ Do you feel more angry or anxious after seeing certain content online?
- ❒ Is there someone you are chatting to online who started as supportive but pushes hateful or extreme ideas as though they are "normal" or "no big deal"?
- ❒ Does someone online make you feel "chosen" but only if you agree with them?
- ❒ Is someone online saying violence is a form of justice or defence?
- ❒ Is someone online pushing you to believe that cruelty is "for the greater good"?

If you answered **"Yes"** to any of the above, you are at risk of participating in hate speech and becoming radicalised.

How does technology make hate speech and radicalisation worse for young people?

Daw's story shows that hate speech and radicalisation don't spread by accident. They're often pushed by the technology teens use every day. What started as him watching content that simply matched his curiosity quickly turned into something much darker, not because he went looking for it, but because the platforms kept feeding him more of the same.

The algorithms promote radicalisation by continuously feeding you with content

Social media platforms use algorithms, which are computer programmes, to determine the content you see next when you scroll through your social media screens. These algorithms look at what you click, how long you watch something, and what you like or comment on, and then select content that is similar to what you've viewed before.

These recommendation algorithms prioritise content that is more extreme, sensational, or controversial because they are driven by engagement metrics such as clicks, views, comments, likes, and shares. Recommendation algorithms reward provocative content that is likely to draw strong emotional reactions, such as fear, shock, anger, and outrage.

Avoid feeling trapped in a "filter bubble", which can occur when the recommendation algorithm continues to show you content that matches your past behaviour or beliefs. The problem with this is that you will see similar ideas and views over and over. In social media, birds of a feather flock together.

The "filter bubble" can easily turn into an "echo chamber", which is when a group of users reinforces each other's views, often pushing for hateful and radical content. Thus, rather than the recommendation algorithm steering you away from harmful content, it can guide you towards increasingly hateful and radicalised content over time.

If you watched moderately controversial content, because these recommendation algorithms privilege interaction, they gradually turn it into extreme or radicalised content. To protect yourself from viewing what you always want to view, you need to deceive the recommendation algorithm by following different kinds of accounts, deliberately seeking content that challenges your thinking, or just flicking through the feed (fast scrolling) to rebalance it. You can also delete your watch history and search history. Some social media apps, like TikTok, let you indicate the content you are not interested in.

AI is being used to track and attack problematic content

On the flip side, social media platforms use AI tools to scan for and detect hateful and extremist content. These AI tools often look for patterns in the text, such as certain words, words that often go together, semantic features, or even behavioural signals. Machine learning tools can now identify insults targeting someone's race, religion, or gender. Social media filters can either hide it, blur it, or send it to human moderators. Needless to say, some harmful content can still slip through.

Don't assume that just because a video or post has not been taken down yet, it is safe to watch or view. Social media platforms also employ human moderators who review content flagged by other users or AI tools and either remove it, limit its visibility, or add a warning. To protect yourself from harmful content, unfollow accounts that make you feel uncomfortable, avoid clicking on extreme content, and report such content so it gets blocked.

Use settings and filters to take a proactive approach towards viewing content

Most social media platforms include features that let you filter out certain words or phrases to prevent exposure to hateful messages. On YouTube, this feature is called "Restricted Mode", and on Google it is called "Safe Search". Use such features to stop certain content from appearing in your feed. Use the "Report" button when you come across extremist content or rhetoric that incites violence against individuals or groups. Reporting such content alerts human moderators to take action. As advised in previous chapters, make your account private. Doing this will prevent strangers from messaging you directly, commenting on your posts, or sharing their posts with you.

Radicals use technology to create the "us against them" view

Radicals live by the rule "divide and conquer". After dividing people into groups, they move to establishing their credibility with the groups they target. Once this is achieved, they progress to communicating their ideology, explaining where they differ from others, and providing the "justification" for their thinking, which they often back up with "evidence". Radical groups can invoke several narratives to win the sympathy of vulnerable individuals, but the online radicalisation discourse appeals especially to personal grievances; in fact, invoking personal grievances is the first step in the radicalisation process.

They can also use other measures to garner sympathy, such as a shared identity rooted in a perception of victimhood. They post content that exploits fear, anger, or injustice to elicit a reaction. To protect yourself, question the reason why this content appeared in your feed. If the content invites you to choose them over another group, or uses slurs to describe the other group, then that is a red flag.

You should also question the motive of the person who posted the content:

- ☑ Are they posting for views, or to provoke, or to persuade?
- ☑ If the content is trying to make you angry, fearful, or suspicious, then pause and reflect. You should check the source.
- ☑ Is the source a reputable news organisation, academic institution, government, or well-known community?
- ☑ Is it a social media page maintained by an anonymous account?
- ☑ Does the content cite facts, data, or links to credible sources or reports?

If the content is mostly emotional, makes baseless claims, and uses slogans, then you should avoid it.

What to do if you have experienced hate speech or radicalisation online

Daw didn't realise at first how far things had shifted. What began as casual scrolling slowly changed the way he thought and felt. If you've experienced hate speech or found yourself pulled towards extreme ideas online, you're not alone, and there are practical steps you can take to regain control and protect yourself.

1 Pause all online interactions and step back from viewing content

When you realise you've been caught up in hateful or extreme content, the first thing to do is hit pause, literally and mentally. Stop replying, stop posting, and step away from the accounts, videos, or chats that have been pulling you in. The more you keep looking, the harder it is to break free, because the content is designed to keep you hooked. Taking a step back gives your brain space to reset and think clearly, without the constant pressure of persuasive messages.

> **Legal tip**: While you may come across a lot of material on the internet that offends you, a small proportion of it is actually illegal. Hate material online is recorded by police as a "hate crime" when it meets the legal criteria of a crime committed with hate motivation.

2 Support others online

When people who witness hate, racism, or prejudice speak out against it, it makes the person being targeted feel supported. It can make the person being hateful reconsider their behaviour. Don't put yourself at risk. But if it is safe to do so, speak up and stand with the victim. Even a simple gesture can be powerful.

If you see someone being targeted with hate speech or pulled towards radical ideas online, don't just scroll past; it's not enough to say, "that's not my problem". Staying silent can make the person feel even more isolated, which is exactly what predators want. You don't have to confront the perpetrator directly, but you can check-in privately with the person, offer support, and encourage them to talk to a trusted adult. If the content is harmful, report it to the platform and, if necessary, help them save evidence. Even small acts, like reminding someone they're not alone or pointing them towards safe spaces, can disrupt the cycle and make it harder for hate to grow.

If someone you know is at risk of radicalisation, ask for advice as soon as possible from government websites. This risk is serious and can result in significant mental harm to the person you know. Every country has a government website for support with advice on what you can do if you know someone who is being radicalised or participating in hate speech.

> **Search online for** "[Your country] online radicalisation support"; "[Your country] help for experiencing hate speech online"

3 Save copies of everything

If you've been targeted by hate speech or pulled into radical content online, don't just delete it; save it. Take screenshots, record usernames, URLs, and keep copies of messages, posts, or videos. This evidence can help you explain what happened to a trusted adult, school staff, or law enforcement authorities, and it's important if the situation needs to be reported. Make sure you store it somewhere safe, like a private folder or cloud storage, and don't share it publicly, as that could spread the harmful content further. Saving proof isn't about holding on to negativity; it's about protecting yourself and helping others stop the same thing from happening again.

When saving information, ensure you keep track of the context. Write down what happened before and after the incident. Include details like what was said, who was involved, and how you came across it. This helps show the bigger picture.

4 Block and report the person and content

Once you've saved evidence, report the accounts, groups, or posts to the platform. Many social media platforms have dedicated tools to report hate speech and extremism. After reporting, block the accounts so they can't message or target you again. Removing the source is like shutting a window before a storm; it keeps the toxic content out.

If you see online graphic or violent extremist material or content that supports, directs, or glorifies extremist actions, report it using anonymous online reporting tools, as each country has its own government sites to monitor and track these complaints.

> **Search online for government sites in most countries where you can report extremist content, such as:**
>
> United Kingdom: https://actearly.uk/advice/staying-safe-online/
>
> United Kingdom: https://www.report-it.org.uk/reporting_internet_hate_crime
>
> Australia: https://www.nationalsecurity.gov.au/what-can-i-do/report-suspicious-behaviour/national-security-hotline-online-report
>
> United States: https://www.dhs.gov/see-something-say-something

If the content you've seen or received includes threats of violence, plans for attacks, instructions on making weapons, or encourages you (or others) to harm people or property, involve the police. This isn't "telling on someone or snitching", it's protecting yourself, the people you care about, and others from real danger. Radicalisation and hate speech can cross the line into criminal activity fast, especially if someone is trying to recruit you or pressure you into performing illegal acts. Keep the evidence, tell a trusted adult immediately, and report it to the police. Your safety and the safety of others is more important than staying silent.

The following are indicators of when you should report something to the police:

- ☑ If someone threatens to harm you, others, or damage property
- ☑ If you see plans or instructions for violence or illegal activities
- ☑ If you're being pressured or recruited to commit a crime
- ☑ If you receive messages encouraging self-harm or suicide

Remember: If you're worried that reporting hate speech or radicalisation online might get you in trouble, remember that authorities want to help keep you safe, not punish you for speaking up. Reporting shows responsibility and can protect you from harm. It's always better to get help early than to stay silent and risk things getting worse.

Myth:	If I report something about hate speech or radicalisation, I might get in trouble or even be prosecuted.
Fact:	Reporting shows you're responsible and trying to stay safe. Authorities want to protect you, not punish you for asking for help.
Myth:	If I tell on someone, I'll be labelled a "snitch" or get targeted.
Fact:	Your safety comes first. Reporting can stop harmful behaviour before it hurts more people, and there are ways to keep your identity private and information completely anonymous.
Myth:	It's better to stay quiet and handle it myself.
Fact:	Hate speech and radicalisation can quickly get worse without help. Speaking up early can protect you and others.

5 Reach out for support and focus on positive content

Don't try to deal with it all on your own. Talk to someone like a parent, older sibling, school counsellor, or trusted friend who can help you process what's going on. You don't need to share every detail right away; just explaining that you've been exposed to or drawn into harmful content is enough to start. Having someone outside the situation can help you see it more clearly and stop the cycle before it pulls you in deeper. Remember, this isn't about getting in trouble; it's about getting support so you can get back to being yourself.

When you step away from radical or hateful spaces, there's an empty space in your feed and your mind. Replace it with accounts, videos, or podcasts that encourage kindness, critical thinking, and diverse perspectives. Your brain naturally adjusts to what you consume, so feeding it healthy content makes it easier to stay grounded.

Conclusion

Hate speech and extremist content are prevalent online and can influence young minds. This chapter helps teens recognise and avoid harmful content while promoting respectful digital interactions. It also explores how extremist groups advance their agenda and use personal grievances to recruit individuals online. It identifies early warning signs, intervention strategies, and how to prevent radicalisation. Social media platforms use recommendation algorithms that promote engagement. Content that provokes fear, shock, anger, and outrage gets pushed aggressively, so keep an eye on your social media feed to ensure you are not trapped in a "filter bubble" or worse, an "echo chamber". This chapter offers some practical steps to avoid exposure to hate speech or victimhood, as well as extremism or radicalisation.

Key terms

- Hate speech
- Radicalisation
- Terrorism
- Counter-terrorism
- Extremist
- Encrypted chat
- Propaganda
- Filter bubble
- Echo chamber
- Algorithmic radicalisation
- Online repetition
- Divide and conquer
- Hate groups
- Radical influencers
- Fast scrolling
- Ideology
- Victimhood

Bibliography

Australian Bureau of Statistics. (2025, September 15). *Online safety*. https://www.abs.gov.au/statistics/measuring-what-matters/measuring-what-matters-themes-and-indicators/secure/online-safety

Australian Federal Police. (2024, December 20). *Concerns over children accessing extremist material online*. https://www.afp.gov.au/news-centre/media-release/concerns-over-children-accessing-extremist-material-online

Barton, G. (2024, December 6). *Rates of youth radicalisation are climbing in Australia and abroad. Here's what to look out for*. The Conversation. https://theconversation.com/rates-of-youth-radicalisation-are-climbing-in-australia-and-abroad-heres-what-to-look-out-for-245459

Brooks, L. (2025, August 1). *Far-right extremists using games platforms to radicalise teenagers, report warns*. The Guardian. https://www.theguardian.com/politics/2025/jul/31/far-right-extremists-games-platforms-radicalise-teenagers-report

Edelman on behalf of Microsoft Australia. (2025, February 11). *Two thirds of Australian teens experienced online risk last year, according to new research from Microsoft*. Medianet News Hub. https://newshub.medianet.com.au/2025/02/two-thirds-of-australian-teens-experienced-online-risk-last-year-according-to-new-research-from-microsoft/87035

eSafety Commissioner. (2020). *Online hate speech* [Report]. https://www.esafety.gov.au/sites/default/files/2020-01/Hate%20speech-Report.pdf?v=1780785110791

eSafety Commissioner. (2024, September 6). *Online hate, bullying and violence*. https://www.esafety.gov.au/research/young-people-social-cohesion/online-hate-bullying-violence

eSafety Commissioner. (2026, February 10). *Online hate*. https://www.esafety.gov.au/young-people/online-hate

eSafety Commissioner. (2026, June 4). *Snapshot: Seen online hate*. Australian Government. https://www.esafety.gov.au/research/the-online-experiences-of-children-in-australia/snapshot-seen-online-hate

Europol. (2025). *European Union terrorism situation and trend report 2025 (EU TE-SAT)*. Publications Office of the European Union. https://www.europol.europa.eu/cms/sites/default/files/documents/EU_TE-SAT_2025.pdf

Feiam, A. (2024, December 20). *Urgent warning for parents as horrifying trend among kids emerges online*. News.com.au. https://www.news.com.au/technology/online/urgent-warning-for-parents-as-horrifying-trend-among-kids-emerges-online/news-story/a574d3f67ff6e39eb00483fa8f7920af

Flood, M., & Keddie, A. (2026). Inspiration, advocate, hypocrite or predator? Young men's diverse views of Andrew Tate. *Gender and Education*, 1–18. https://doi.org/10.1080/09540253.2026.2644260

Goel, V., Sahnan, D., Dutta, S., Bandhakavi, A., & Chakraborty, T. (2023). *Hatemongers ride on echo chambers to escalate hate speech diffusion* (arXiv:2302.02479). arXiv. https://doi.org/10.48550/arXiv.2302.02479

Grant, J. I. (2021, April 29). *Online extremist movements and radicalism in Australia*. eSafety Commissioner. https://www.esafety.gov.au/newsroom/blogs/online-extremist-movements-and-radicalism-in-australia

Greene, A. (2024, December 6). *Five Eyes security agencies take unprecedented step to fight youth terrorism threat*. ABC News. https://www.abc.net.au/news/2024-12-06/five-eyes-nations-issue-warn-rising-youth-radicalisation/104692476

Hindustan Times. (2025, April 13). *Radicalised at 12: Alarming rise of child terror suspects in Europe*. https://www.hindustantimes.com/world-news/radicalised-at-12-alarming-rise-of-child-terror-suspects-in-europe-101744529391338.html

Kardefelt Winther, D., Stoilova, M., Büchi, M., Twesigye, R., Smahel, D., Bedrosová, M., Kvardová, N., & Livingstone, S. (2023, July). *Children's exposure to hate messages and violent images online*. UNICEF Innocenti – Global Office of Research and Foresight. https://www.unicef.org/innocenti/media/2621/file/UNICEF-Children-Exposure-Hate-Violence-Online.pdf

Koh, F. (2025, July 29). *ISD terrorism threat, Israel-Palestine, far-right extremism, ISIS, al-Qaeda, social media, youths*. Channel NewsAsia. https://www.channelnewsasia.com/singapore/isd-terrorism-threat-israel-palestine-far-right-extremism-isis-al-qaeda-social-media-youths-5262646

Leicester, J. (2025, April 13). *Teen exposed to extremist content in France*. AP News. https://apnews.com/article/4888bab2d10502edadf787d419d45b5b

Oksanen, A., Hawdon, J., Holkeri, E., Näsi, M., & Räsänen, P. (2014). Exposure to online hate among young social media users. *Soul of Society: A Focus on the Lives of Children & Youth* (Sociological Studies of Children and Youth, Volume 18). https://doi.org/10.1108/S1537-466120140000018021.

One Giant Leap. (2025, May 20). *Facing the digital storm: Online hate in 2025*. https://www.insights.onegiantleap.com/blogs/facing-the-digital-storm-online-hate-in-2025

Saplagio, A. (2025, February 17). *Microsoft report: 64% of Australian teens faced online risks in 2024*. Comms Room. https://commsroom.co/microsoft-report-64-of-australian-teens-faced-online-risks-in-2024

Sun, D. (2025, July 30). *Online platforms have halved time it takes for Singaporeans to be self-radicalised: ISD*. The Straits Times. https://www.straitstimes.com/singapore/online-platforms-chat-groups-have-halved-time-it-takes-for-singaporeans-to-be-self-radicalised-isd

UNICEF Innocenti. (2023, July). *Children's exposure to hate messages and violent images online*. https://www.unicef.org/innocenti/documents/childrens-exposure-hate-messages-and-violent-images-online

Whittaker, J. (2023). *RAN policy support: Online radicalisation* [Report]. European Commission.https://home-affairs.ec.europa.eu/system/files/2023-11/RAN-online-radicalisation_en.pdf

Wikipedia contributors. (n.d.). *Algorithmic radicalization*. Wikipedia. Retrieved June 6, 2026, from https://en.wikipedia.org/wiki/Algorithmic_radicalization

Wikipedia contributors. (n.d.). *Far-right usage of social media*. Wikipedia. Retrieved June 6, 2026, from https://en.wikipedia.org/wiki/Far right_usage_of_social_media

Wikipedia contributors. (n.d.). *Online youth radicalization*. Wikipedia. Retrieved June 6, 2026, from https://en.wikipedia.org/wiki/Online_youth_radicalization

Wong, K. (2024, December 6). *Aus teens being pushed towards violence online*. The New Daily. https://www.thenewdaily.com.au/life/tech/2024/12/06/online-violence-australia-radical

Yorke, H. (2024, December 9). *Nearly half of young men like Andrew Tate, extremism tsar warns*. The Times. https://www.thetimes.co.uk/article/nearly-half-of-young-men-like-andrew-tate-extremism-tsar-warns-0mb9cfhcm

9 How to avoid fake news and online misinformation

Today, Samuel will find out his fate. He is at home sitting on the sofa with his mum in the living room in front of a laptop. He is attending his court proceedings via a video link. As the judge began the process of reading the verdict, Samuel's mother held his hands tightly. "How did I get here?" Samuel thought to himself. His mum is immunodeficient. When Covid-19 hit, Samuel became extremely worried about her. He knew his mum would be more vulnerable to the severe outcomes from the virus, but did not know how she could protect herself from falling victim to the virus. His mum's doctor confirmed that even though she was vaccinated, her immune system may not produce strong protection. To educate himself on how to prevent his mum from contracting COVID-19, Samuel went to social media, especially Facebook and YouTube, for medical advice. Sadly, his worst fears were confirmed. Like most of the people in his town, his mum contracted the virus and immediately developed severe respiratory issues. Seeing his mum taken into hospital and placed in intensive care made him develop intense feelings of anger about COVID-19. As Samuel doomscrolled through Facebook for information on immunodeficiency and COVID, he came across mounting evidence that COVID was spread by 5G towers. His thought that this was "a stupid idea" was interrupted by the knock on the front door. "Quick," his best mate screamed. "Where are we going?" Samuel asked. "We are taking matters into our own hands," his friend responded as they got into the car. "I have been keeping an eye on the 5G tower on Gap Road for a while. I have never seen a car pass by that road after 9 pm. I am setting this 5G tower on fire tonight. You can thank me later," his friend said. "Are you insane? I am not doing that. Stop the car!" Samuel yelled. Unfortunately for them, someone in a car saw the friend set the 5G tower on fire and then flee in a car that Samuel was driving. The police instantly recognised the duo in the dashcam footage the car driver handed over and sent for them to attend the police station for questioning.

DOI: 10.4324/9781003681731-10

The rise of digital deception

False and misleading information has become a widespread challenge in the digital age, especially for teenagers. A 2023 report found that 51% of teens encounter misleading or false information online every day, yet only 26% feel confident in their ability to distinguish fact from fiction.

In 2025, research showed that a large majority of people encountered misinformation regularly, with around 72% of adults saying the spread of false information online was a major threat to society. Those who use digital platforms reported encountering some form of misinformation, most often on apps like Instagram, X, and TikTok. Among Australian teenagers, 44% were exposed to misinformation and disinformation in the past year, making it one of the most common online risks they face. Among younger internet users globally, research finds that around 35% of teens say they've been misled by fake content online, and about 22% admit they have shared something they later learned was fake. These statistics highlight how frequently teens and adults alike encounter false or misleading information, underscoring the importance of developing strong critical thinking and digital literacy skills.

After 17-year-old school football star Austin Metcalf was fatally stabbed at a track meet in Texas, misinformation rapidly spread across social media about what had actually happened. Following the tragic incident, fake social media accounts impersonating law enforcement and medical officials posted false claims, including that Metcalf died of a drug overdose or as the result of "mutual combat", rather than from the confirmed stabbing. These fabricated posts amplified confusion, hurt the family's grieving process, and diverted attention from the actual incident and its consequences.

Research conducted at a hospital found that two-thirds of teens take health advice from social media, and that much of it is unverified and promoted by creators without medical credentials. Misinformation about dieting, exercise, and wellness trends, often lacking scientific evidence, contributes to confusion and unhealthy decision-making among teens, particularly girls who tend to receive a disproportionate amount of health content in their feeds.

AI-generated content is a key contributor

The rapid growth of AI-generated content has made the spread of misinformation far more complex and difficult to control. Research shows that a rapidly growing proportion of online content is generated or assisted by AI, including text, images, videos, and chatbot responses. A 2023 study found that AI tools, including chatbots and deepfake generators, were used to produce hundreds of fake news articles and highly realistic synthetic videos, many of which circulated widely before being detected or removed. Unlike traditional media, AI-generated content can be created quickly, cheaply, and at a massive scale, often without any human editorial oversight. As a result, misleading or false information can spread faster than fact-checkers and platforms can respond.

What is adversarial AI?

Adversarial AI involves deliberately manipulating or feeding false or misleading information into algorithms, allowing AI systems to learn, amplify, or spread misinformation at scale. This often makes fake content appear more credible, personalised, and harder for people to detect.

In 2024, an investigation revealed that hundreds of AI-generated news and information websites were publishing misleading or false content on a large scale, often without human supervision. At the same time, many teenagers regularly encounter AI-generated summaries, images, and videos online without realising they were created by AI. Because AI tools can produce content that appears confident, emotional, and highly convincing, even when it is inaccurate or entirely false, it has become increasingly difficult for everyone, but especially teens, to distinguish factual information from misinformation. This raises the risk that misinformation can influence beliefs, emotions, and real-world decisions before there is time to stop, question, or verify what is being viewed.

Under media regulations, online advertisements must comply with media codes that require clear labelling. This means all ads should be visibly identified using labels such as "Ad", "Advertisement", "Branded Content", "Promoted", "Sponsored", or "Paid Partnership" to ensure transparency for viewers. A study found that two-thirds of high school students couldn't differentiate between a legitimate news article and an advertisement when evaluating online information. This illustrates how easily misinformation can shape young people's opinions, political views, and even health decisions. Research further suggests that younger generations, including Gen Z, are more susceptible to fake news than older adults. This vulnerability stems from their high digital media engagement combined with the increasingly convincing nature of synthetic content.

What is the difference between misinformation and disinformation?

The difference is in the intent of sharing the information:

- *Misinformation* is false or inaccurate information: "getting the facts wrong"
- *Disinformation* is false information which is deliberately intended to mislead: "intentionally misstating the facts"

In Australia, over 80% of parents express concern about their children's exposure to harmful AI-generated content, a worry shared by many teens themselves. A 2024 US survey found that 59% of teenagers aged 13–18 are concerned about AI-generated misinformation, while 58% are worried about deepfakes. These concerns were ranked just below healthcare access and affordability and above other critical issues such as social inequality and climate change, which demonstrates the growing impact of AI-driven misinformation on youth perceptions.

Deepfakes are a growing concern

The rapid rise of deepfake technology has triggered crises in schools. Reports show that most deepfake content involving students is pornographic, with girls and young women being disproportionately affected. These AI-generated images and videos are often shared without consent and can spread quickly through social media and messaging apps, causing serious emotional harm. Beyond individual incidents, AI-generated content can also reinforce harmful stereotypes, promote false narratives, and distort social norms. Over time, this exposure can shape teenagers' values, self-image, and behaviour, contributing to lasting psychological and social damage.

Deepfake technology is no longer rare or experimental. It is increasingly being used to target young people in harmful ways. Research shows that around one in four teenagers has seen a sexually explicit deepfake online, often involving classmates, people they know, or other minors. In addition, about one in eight teens knows someone who has been targeted, and a smaller but significant number report being victims themselves.

A 13-year-old girl in Louisiana was ridiculed and traumatised after boys at her school shared AI-generated explicit images of her and her friends on social media. Initially, she was expelled despite not being at fault. The legal system ultimately charged those responsible for disseminating the deepfake images, but the emotional impact on the victim, including anxiety and depression requiring therapy, highlighted how deepfake misuse can hurt teens and overwhelm school policies.

The impact of fake news and misinformation online is severe

Exposure to fake news and misinformation doesn't just affect what teens believe. It can influence their emotions, behaviours, and trust in real information. Research shows that many young people struggle to tell fact from fiction. These experiences can lead to severe psychological impacts, including anxiety, shame, fear of social judgement, and long-term damage to self-esteem. Because fake content is designed to look real and spread rapidly, victims often feel powerless to control its effects. Experts warn that teenagers are particularly vulnerable due to their high online engagement, the fact that they are still developing critical thinking skills, and the increasing sophistication of AI-generated content.

In one study, only about 11% of 11–17-year-olds could reliably identify genuine online content, meaning most teens are vulnerable to believing misleading information without realising. Another study focusing on health information found that 41% of teenagers could not distinguish between true and fake online health messages, which can lead to poor decisions about health and well-being. Frequent exposure to fake news on social media has also been linked to higher levels of stress and anxiety, with research indicating that teens who encounter misinformation more often are more likely to experience negative emotional effects. Because misinformation often appears repeatedly and in familiar formats, teens may begin to accept falsehoods as truth, undermining their trust in credible sources and making it harder to make informed choices.

How online media uses manipulative techniques to influence you

Samuel's emotional state made him vulnerable to fake news and misinformation. The psychological tactics being used on him online were powerful enough to turn a usually thoughtful and sensible person into someone unable to think critically for himself. Samuel was completely unaware that he was being manipulated into thinking, feeling, and doing things based on false information spread online.

Psychological tactics used online to spread fake news and misinformation are powerful because they exploit the human desire for social validation, emotional satisfaction, and feeling like you belong. Together, they create an environment where misinformation can spread quickly, become entrenched, and even shape real-world decisions. These strategies are used to capture attention, manipulate emotions, and drive engagement. These online information-sharing groups often exploit cognitive and emotional responses that can affect decision-making, beliefs, and behaviours. Understanding these manipulative techniques is critical for resilience against misinformation.

Social validation makes you want to fit in

Social media platforms and news outlets leverage others' behaviour to influence individual decisions. The more likes, shares, or comments something gets, the more likely others are to trust and engage with it. Content that achieves more attention is perceived as more credible or valuable, even if it's misleading. The content sharers use tactics, such as social support, to reinforce engagement behaviours. The desire to fit in or be part of a group can lead users, especially teens, to share or believe information based on its popularity rather than its accuracy.

What to look for to determine when online content is designed to achieve social validation:

- ☑ Large amounts of likes, comments, and shares
- ☑ Influencer or a well-known person endorsing the content
- ☑ Comments that overwhelmingly agree with or reinforce the message shared
- ☑ Trending hashtags or posts that announce their own popularity
- ☑ Asking for comments and reciprocating with likes or additional comments

Automation bias shapes what you believe

Algorithms exploit automation bias by presenting information that becomes an anchor, shaping what teenagers believe before they have a chance to question it. There is a natural tendency for people to favour information that confirms their pre-existing beliefs and ignore information that differs from what they know. Algorithms continue to show content that aligns with something you have engaged with, which continues to reinforce information you may be biased towards.

Social media posts or news stories often present misleading or emotionally charged headlines that serve as anchors. This means that the first information you see (the anchor) influences your perception of subsequent information. Even if the subsequent content provides more context or refutes the initial claim, you are likely to rely on the first piece of information you encountered. Misinformation thrives in this environment, as you are less likely to critically challenge content that resonates with your own initial reaction to it.

They use sensationalism, clickbait, and emotional triggers to get you hooked

Headlines and content in fake news and misinformation are usually sensationalised to provoke curiosity and drive clicks. By using emotionally charged or exaggerated headlines, outlets manipulate you into clicking on articles to falsely increase the popularity of content. These headlines may be inaccurate or misleading, but they are designed to lure you towards reading seemingly popular, sensational information. This clickbait encourages addictive behaviours, where you continually return for more stimulation, often prioritising entertainment or sensationalism over accuracy.

Platforms capitalise on the fear of not fitting in or fear of missing out (FOMO) to keep you engaged, creating a sense of urgency or anxiety. This emotional manipulation is often driven by narratives that focus on what everyone else agrees with and time-limited offers that make people feel like they must respond quickly. This fear can lead you to consume large amounts of information quickly, without critically assessing its validity. This emotional tactic increases impulsivity, making you more susceptible to believing fake news or misinformation.

Online content is also often crafted to trigger strong emotions such as shock, anger, fear, sadness, or happiness. If content evokes an emotional response or triggers it, then it usually bypasses critical thinking, and you are more likely to share, comment, and remember it. Emotionally charged posts are usually based on what people fear or topics that create a divide between groups, which can lead to viral misinformation.

Examples of headlines that indicate fake news or misinformation

Sensationalism	* SHOCKING, the truth the government doesn't want you to know! * You won't believe what this doctor just exposed about vaccines!
Clickbait	* Celebs who aged terribly – #7 will break your heart * This is the real reason why your school is failing you
Emotional Triggers	* This sick puppy was left to die until one stranger stepped in * If you don't share this, you don't care about children in need

By using selective exposure, it targets your personalisation bias

In the online world, "echo chambers" and "filter bubbles" play major roles in spreading and reinforcing fake news and misinformation. Filter bubbles limit what teenagers are exposed to, while echo chambers reinforce those ideas until they feel like they are the only truth. These effects are driven by social media algorithms and personal browsing habits, which shape the content users see online by showing them more content that they have viewed or engaged with.

An online echo chamber occurs when people mostly engage with content and communities that reflect their own views. When you repeatedly see the same opinions and ideas, it creates the illusion that they are universally accepted or factual. For example, when Samuel started watching videos about vaccine scepticism on YouTube, he was likely quickly recommended more of the same content, eventually becoming immersed in an environment where false information is constantly echoed and rarely challenged.

A filter bubble is created by algorithms that personalise content feeds based on user activity, such as likes, shares, watch history, and searches. On all online platforms, you are shown content tailored to your preferences, which can unintentionally shield you from credible sources or diverse viewpoints. For instance, if Samuel repeatedly watches or clicks on conspiracy-related content (e.g., "5G causes illness" or "COVID is a hoax"), the algorithm may stop showing reliable news sources and instead reinforce the same misinformation.

These online dynamics trap you in a self-reinforcing loop, in which misinformation is repeatedly presented as fact and critical thinking is discouraged.

Because content in an echo chamber or filter bubble often appears popular (with thousands of likes, shares, or comments), it can gain false credibility through social validation, further blurring the line between what is true and what is not.

Samuel fell victim to emotional manipulation, confirmation bias, and repetition-based misinformation. His fear and anxiety over his mother's illness made him emotionally vulnerable, leading him to search for answers on social media platforms that often promote sensational, emotionally triggering, and conspiratorial content. As he doomscrolled, the algorithm amplified emotionally charged and misleading information, such as the false link between COVID-19 and 5G towers. Repeated exposure to this misinformation, paired with his emotional state, lowered his scepticism and critical thinking. This repeated exposure to incorrect information increased his susceptibility to false beliefs, even when he was initially unsure about the content. His experience shows how fear, repetition, social proof, echo chambers, and algorithmic exposure can converge to influence beliefs and real-world offline actions.

Check-in: Before you trust something you see online, consider the following:

- ❒ Is the source clear and credible, or anonymous and unfamiliar?
- ❒ Does the information make you feel angry, scared, shocked, or outraged right away?
- ❒ Can you find the same information on trusted news sites or official sources?
- ❒ Are there facts, quotes, or data, *OR* just opinions, screenshots, or claims with no proof?
- ❒ Do headlines contain ALL CAPS or extreme claims saying you must share with others?
- ❒ Does the image, video, or audio look unusually perfect, edited, or AI-generated?

If any of the above might be answered with a **"Yes"**, you should ensure that you follow the steps to critically assess the information before considering it as factual.

How to critically assess information you see online

Samuel's experience shows how easily anyone can be pulled in by information that looks real, confident, and convincing online. The posts he watched were shared widely, backed by strong opinions, and repeated so often that they began to feel true, even when they weren't. This is why learning how to critically assess the information you see online is so important. Fake news and misinformation don't always come from obvious sources. They often appear in videos, comments, memes, or AI-generated content designed to trigger emotion rather than thought. Knowing how to pause, question, and verify information provided by technology helps ensure you don't fall victim to online misinformation.

Always follow the cybersecurity principle zero trust

The zero-trust principle assumes no user or device can be trusted; so never trust, always verify. Before we address how to critically assess information you see online, let us first unpack what we mean by critically assessing information.

Critically assessing information means systematically evaluating the information you are seeing, rather than just accepting it at face value. This can involve questioning everything you see online, including:

- ☑ Who created this information and why?
- ☑ What is their motive or agenda?
- ☑ Do they have the qualifications and expertise (credentials)?
- ☑ Did they back up their information with evidence?
- ☑ When was the information created, and is it still relevant?

You should also examine the source of the information, ensuring it is credible, and, if it references other sources, check the links to those sources. As you go through this information, look for flaws and inconsistencies as well as completeness to ensure it has not been cherry-picked or taken out of context. Likewise, you should consider your own biases so as not to naively believe anything you see simply because it aligns with your expectations.

Use cross-referencing to validate information from credible sources

You should always cross-reference this information with credible sources that are authoritative on the topic. Imagine you are lying in bed, scrolling through TikTok, when a video appears showing a plane with its wings on fire, plummeting towards a building you recognise. As the sound of screaming in the video grows louder, your heart begins to race uncontrollably because you realise that your dad could be working in that building. But before you panic or call him, pause and check whether the video is real. A plane crash would be breaking news, so first, turn on the TV or visit a trusted news site like abc.net.au/news to confirm the facts.

Always start with the assumption that the information cannot be trusted

Back to the question: How can you critically assess information you see online? Following the principle of zero trust, you should always approach anything you see on social media as inherently untrustworthy until proven otherwise.

There are several reliable tools and easy-to-follow methods that you can use to check if a video, for example, you have seen on a social media platform like TikTok, YouTube, or Instagram, is real or fake. You could use reverse search tools, metadata checkers, and fact-checking platforms. Let us look at some of those methods in more detail. If the content is important, examine it as a forensic investigator would, checking carefully for signs that it might be edited, manipulated, or misleading.

Train yourself to spot fake videos

First, check who uploaded the video. Is the account real and trustworthy? You can determine whether the account is fake and untrustworthy by checking if the username (social media handle) is unusual (e.g., made up of random characters) or if the bio is missing. If either of these conditions is met, then this is a red flag.

Second, investigate whether the profile photo has been copied from the internet. You can do this by doing a reverse image search on the profile photo. If the profile photo appears on multiple websites or belongs to someone else, then this video can't be considered trustworthy.

Third, take a look at the account's network size. If the user has very few followers, that is, very few people follow them, then treat this account with suspicion. If the account only ever reposts, reshares, re-tweets, or clips someone else's content without posting any original content, then the account could be a bot uploading content on behalf of someone or a new account trying to monetise from someone else's content. In comparison, authentic accounts, such as those for official news channels or well-known influencers, tend to have detailed profiles, many followers, and verified badges.

Fourth, check the uploader of the content to see if they have been posting regularly over time. If the account is brand new, with fewer posts, then treat it with caution. You can also try to locate the original video to ensure you are not looking at a modified version of the same. You can do this by copying the video's caption or an important phrase that appeared in the video and searching for it using Google or AI agents. You should also look at the context associated with the video content. Take note of the time the video was posted. When I visit YouTube, I often encounter videos of highlights of soccer matches that have not been played yet. The uploaders of these videos show highlights of old matches a day before the match is played to trick soccer enthusiasts into clicking on their videos so they can get more views. For this reason, it is important to pay attention to the time the video is uploaded.

Be aware of how censorship, deplatforming, and content moderation increase misinformation

While censorship, deplatforming, and content moderation are intended to reduce harmful content online, they can sometimes unintentionally fuel the spread of misinformation. When social media platforms remove posts or ban users, it can create a sense of secrecy or suppression, making false claims seem more credible to certain audiences. This often leads people to seek out censored content on less-regulated platforms, which in turn makes misinformation spread. In some cases, content warnings or takedowns trigger you to double down on your beliefs rather than question them. These dynamics can strengthen echo chambers, increase distrust in authorities, and ultimately amplify the very misinformation they aim to control.

Train yourself to detect AI-generated content and deepfakes

AI is bound to produce deepfakes that are almost impossible to distinguish from the real. You should train your eye to spot the red flags. AI-created deepfakes contain subtle mistakes. Using videos again as an example of typical social media content, ask yourself: Is the video quality clear? Does the audio match lip movement? Is there a glitch or a twitch somewhere in the video? Also, keep an eye on the eyes in a video, and the jaw movements. Notice whether the eyes blink normally or naturally, or if they do not. If they blink too little or too much, then this glitch is a clue that it is a deepfake.

The same goes for jaw movements; if the face shifts unnaturally or if there is misalignment in the movement of the head, eyes, and lips, then it is not a human face, because a human face is perfectly aligned. A mismatch between lip movement and speech in a video is a clue that the video has been edited. A lack of synchronisation between video and audio is a clear sign that the video is fake. Audio in a video can easily give away if it is fake. Many videos on social media use audio-dubbing (the speech is text-generated). The audio is often monotonous, robotic, and void of human tones. Videos like these are most likely AI-generated.

Verifying the authenticity of content on social media, including videos, is a key skill that everyone should develop in this AI world. Reverse image search is one method you can use to verify the authenticity of images and videos, and there are many free tools out there that you can use to perform reverse image searches, including images.google.com.[1] For example, you can pause a video you want to inspect at a key moment, such as when the airline name is clearly visible, and take a screenshot and upload it to images.google.com. Google may tell you if that image has appeared online. If the search result indicates the exact moment in the video (image) has appeared on a news website or an old video, then the video could be fake.

You can also use AI tools like ChatGPT to help investigate information. For images, try performing a reverse image search with TinEye.com. If you want to get a bit more advanced, the InVID browser extension can break a video into multiple key frames, search each frame across search engines like Google, DuckDuckGo, and Bing, and provide metadata about each frame. On your phone, you can use Google Lens to see if key frames from a video appear elsewhere online. There are also tools like https://ezgif.com/reverse-video and https://www.videoreverser.com/ that allow you to reverse videos to check for edits or inconsistencies.

Use sophisticated search queries to validate information

You can also use Google Hacking (also known as Google Dorking) to carry out sophisticated search queries that will enable you to find exact results. Keywords like site, intext, intitle, before and after, and filetype followed by a colon ":", can pinpoint exact results. Suppose you saw another video of another plane descending at lightning speed. Typing in the Google search box site: abc.net.au plane crash after:2025-07-15 will return results of plane crashes (if any) reported on abc.net.au after 15 July 2025.

The Wayback Machine (Archive.org) is also an indispensable tool for checking past versions of content because the Wayback Machine takes snapshots of online content and makes them available for search. Suppose you visited abc.net.au on 15 July 2025 to watch a video of an Air India plane crash, which occurred on 12 June 2025. Your search for the video using Google Hacking within abc.net.au did not return a link to the video. By entering abc.net.au into the Wayback Machine's URL search box and selecting a snapshot from 12 June 2025 taken after news of the crash began making headlines, you can view the version of the site where the news outlet had just broken the story and included the crash video.

Finally, you can also use Open-Source Intelligence Tools (OSINT) to conduct further research about the source you suspect. You can use TheHarvester to gather emails, names, and social media accounts of individuals (such as video uploaders) from publicly available online sources. You can use Sherlock to check the availability of usernames (for video uploaders) across multiple online platforms. If the world of Open-Source Intelligence excites you, you can use advanced tools like Maltego (Community edition), which is used by private investigators to map relationships between people, images, and websites, allowing you to build a profile of the uploader and the connections they have with other people.

What to do if you have fallen victim to fake news or misinformation

Samuel's story also shows something important: being affected by fake news or misinformation doesn't mean you're careless or unintelligent. It means the technology and content worked the way they were designed to. Misinformation often spreads by tapping into fear, anger, or trust, and it can influence anyone before they realise what's happening. If you've fallen victim to fake news, what matters most is not what you believed at first, but what you do next.

1 Recheck the information using the tools provided earlier and stop engaging

Take a moment to pause when you think you may have interacted with fake news or misinformation. Before reacting or sharing anything further, double- or triple-check the information, especially if your instincts tell you something doesn't feel right. Most importantly, stop engaging with the content. Avoid liking, commenting on, or resharing it, even if you want to argue or correct it. Any interaction can increase its visibility and help it spread to others.

To check whether something is accurate, use reliable and trustworthy sources, as outlined earlier in this chapter, such as:

- ☑ Official government or health websites
- ☑ Respected news organisations with ethical reporting guidelines and standards
- ☑ Independent fact-checking websites (search "list of fact-checking websites" on Wikipedia for a global directory)
- ☑ Talk to parents, caregivers, teachers, or mentors you respect and ask their opinion

2 Take accountability for anything you have interacted with

If you have shared information that could be false or misleading, it's ok. It happens. What you do next is more important:

- Delete any content that could be considered misinformation – this could be reshares, posts, videos, or comments.
- Remove your interactions with false content – such as likes or comments. It's best not to engage at all, even to argue or disagree, as this can still boost content visibility and make it appear trustworthy.
- If needed, follow up with a correction – you could say something like, "I recently shared a post that turned out to be inaccurate. I've looked into it further and want to correct what I shared".

These actions not only stop the spread of misinformation, but also build trust with your friends, family, and followers.

3 Report content and block users

If you encounter misleading or fake content, especially if it's harmful or dangerous, it is important to "report and block":

- **Report**: Use the platform's reporting tools to report the content or account. Most social media platforms allow you to report misinformation under categories such as "false information" or "fake content".
- **Block**: Consider blocking or unfollowing users who repeatedly share false or misleading content. Platforms monitor patterns of reported behaviour, and consistent reports can lead to action being taken against those accounts.

4 Speak up and help others (active bystander)

If you know someone, like a family member or friend, is spreading misinformation, consider talking to them privately. Most people don't deliberately share false information. They may simply be unaware that it is misleading. You can respectfully offer credible sources to help them consider other perspectives.

Just like you would step in if you saw someone putting themselves at risk offline, it is important to do the same online by encouraging people you know to make better choices regarding misinformation.

Conclusion

In an AI world, where AI can be used to create fake and misleading content and also detect that such content is fake and misleading, your default position should be not to trust anything unless proven trustworthy. Watch out for the manipulative online media techniques that can make you lose your guard, such as social validation, algorithmic bias, and sensationalism. Remember, false and misleading information spreads quickly online, influencing beliefs, behaviours, and even real-world decisions. The use of AI has exacerbated this phenomenon. AI has made deepfakes more believable and difficult to dispute. This chapter educates teenagers on how to critically assess information, recognise misinformation and disinformation, and verify sources. It also provides tools to foster digital literacy and analytical thinking, while offering insights into the broader challenges of regulating online misinformation.

Key terms

- Fake news
- Misinformation
- Disinformation
- Adversarial AI
- Chatbots
- Deepfakes
- Social validation
- Automation bias
- Algorithmic biasing
- Anchoring
- Sensationalism
- Clickbait
- Emotional triggers
- Echo chambers
- Filter bubbles
- Censorship
- Deplatforming
- Content moderation
- Zero-trust principle
- Selective exposure
- Personalisation bias

Notes

1 https://www.google.com/imghp.

Bibliography

American Psychological Association. (2023). *Misinformation and disinformation: An expert consensus report* [Report]. https://www.apa.org/pubs/reports/misinformation-consensus-statement.pdf

Australian Communications and Media Authority. (2025, November 24). *Majority of Australians encountering misinformation online.* https://www.acma.gov.au/articles/2025-11/majority-australians-encountering-misinformation-online

Beauvais C. (2022). Fake news: Why do we believe it? *Joint Bone Spine, 89*(4), 105371. https://doi.org/10.1016/j.jbspin.2022.105371

Booth, H. (2024, October 26). *Teenagers and AI risk: What lawmakers need to know.* Time. https://time.com/7098524/teenagers-ai-risk-lawmakers/

Burgelman, S. (2022, August 29). *Teenagers' health influenced by fake messages shared online.* Frontiers. https://www.frontiersin.org/news/2022/08/29/psychology-teenagers-health-fake-messages

Common Sense Media. (2025). *Teens, trust, and technology in the age of AI* [Report]. https://www.commonsensemedia.org/sites/default/files/research/report/teens-trust-and-technology-in-the-age-of-ai_v2_web.pdf

Crane, E. (2025, April 7). *Sick conspiracy theories spread online about slain Texas football star Austin Metcalf's death.* New York Post. https://nypost.com/2025/04/07/us-news/austin-metcalfs-stabbing-death-sparks-sick-conspiracy-theories/

Digital Watch Observatory. (2025, July 23). *Teens struggle to spot misinformation despite daily social media use.* https://dig.watch/updates/teens-struggle-to-spot-misinformation-despite-daily-social-media-use

Donald, B. (2016, November 22). Stanford Graduate School of Education. *Stanford researchers find students have trouble judging the credibility of information online.* https://ed.stanford.edu/news/stanford-researchers-find-students-have-trouble-judging-credibility-information-online

Edelman on behalf of Microsoft Australia. (2025, February 11). *Two-thirds of Australian teens experienced online risk last year, according to new research from Microsoft.* Microsoft. https://newshub.medianet.com.au/2025/02/two-thirds-of-australian-teens-experienced-online-risk-last-year-according-to-new-research-from-microsoft/87035/

Farivar, C. (2025, March 3). *A staggering number of teens personally know someone targeted by deepfake nudes.* Forbes. https://www.forbes.com/sites/cyrusfarivar/2025/03/03/a-staggering-number-of-teens-personally-know-someone-targeted-by-deepfake-nudes/

Fried, I. (2024, August 27). *Exclusive: Chatbots pose unique risks to teens.* Axios. https://www.axios.com/2024/08/27/chatbots-risks-teens-common-sense-media

Girlguiding. (2025, February 11). *One in four teens have seen pornographic deepfakes online.* https://www.girlguiding.org.uk/about-us/press-releases/one-in-four-teens-have-seen-pornographic-deepfakes-online/

Hollingsworth, H., & Brook, J. (2025, December 23). *Boys at her school shared AI-generated, nude images of her. After a fight, she was the one expelled.* Associated Press. https://apnews.com/article/0ead324241cf390e1a7f3378853f23cb

Johar, G. (2025, January 28). *The psychology of fake news: Why people share misinformation.* Columbia Business School, Columbia University. https://business.columbia.edu/research-brief/psychology-of-fake-news-why-people-share-misinformation

Kelly, J. (2024, September 26). *Research finds Gen Z, millennials more vulnerable to fake news.* University of Virginia. https://news.virginia.edu/content/research-finds-gen-z-millennials-more-vulnerable-fake-news

Microsoft. (2024). *Global Online Safety Survey results 2024.* https://cdn-dynmedia-1.microsoft.com/is/content/microsoftcorp/microsoft/final/en-us/microsoft-brand/documents/Global-Online-Safety-Survey-Results-2024.pdf

Mitchell, S. (2025, February 11). *Microsoft survey reveals online risks for Aussie teens.* SecurityBrief Australia. https://securitybrief.com.au/story/microsoft-survey-reveals-online-risks-for-aussie-teens

Nguyen, T.T., Nguyen, D.C., Nguyen, H.T. *et al.* (2025). Exposure to fake news on social media, coping mechanisms, and mental health impact among Vietnamese adolescents and young adults. *Scientific Reports, 15*, 35117. https://doi.org/10.1038/s41598-025-19175-4

Not My Kid. (n.d.). *Children, AI and safety: A guide for Australian parents.* https://notmykid.com.au/children-ai-and-safety-a-guide-for-australian-parents/

Nwoko, H. (2024, July 17). *Social media can be good for Black and Latine youth—If they're digitally literate.* Parents. https://www.parents.com/digital-literacy-for-black-and-latine-youth-8678221

O'Connor, H. NewsGuard. (2024, November). *Watch out: AI "News" sites are on the rise.* https://www.newsguardtech.com/insights/watch-out-ai-news-sites-are-on-the-rise/

Organisation for Economic Co-operation and Development. (n.d.). *Artificial intelligence.* https://www.oecd.org/digital/artificial-intelligence

Pennycook, G., & Rand, D.G. (2021). The psychology of fake news. *Trends in Cognitive Sciences, 25*(5), 388–402. https://doi.org/10.1016/j.tics.2021.02.007

Poushter, J., Fagan, M., Smerkovich, M., & Prozorovsky, A. (2025, August 19). *False information online as a threat.* Pew Research Center. https://www.pewresearch.org/global/2025/08/19/false-information-online-as-a-threat/

Prashnu, V. (2023, December 17). *How AI is making fake news harder to detect.* The Washington Post. https://www.washingtonpost.com/technology/2023/12/17/ai-fake-news-misinformation/

Schmidt, N. (2024, July 23). *Proposed deepfake bill not enough to combat unprecedented crisis.* News.com.au. https://www.news.com.au/technology/online/proposed-deepfake-bill-not-enough-to-combat unprecedented-crisis/news-story/ffb8e5f9a661ef9270b222c5ff4e0dec

Skipper, Y. (2025). 'I'd probably scroll by': An exploration of young people's views on spotting and stopping misinformation. *Children & Society, 39*, 940–949. https://doi.org/10.1111/chso.12962

United Nations Educational, Scientific and Cultural Organization. (2025). *The guidelines for the governance of digital platforms and generative artificial intelligence: Companion document* [Report]. https://unesdoc.unesco.org/ark:/48223/pf0000395825

Walker, T. (2020, January 6). *Students still can't tell fact from fiction on the internet.* Education Week. https://ky.aflcio.org/news/nea-today-students-still-can-t-tell-fact-fiction-internet

Walkim, M. (2025, September 1). *Health misinformation rife on social media, researcher warns.* ABC News. https://www.abc.net.au/news/2025-09-01/health-misinformation-rife-on-social-media-researcher-warns/10569524

10 The risks of online gaming

At the hospital's gaming addiction clinic, Toby, a 13-year-old boy, was the youngest in the room. As his turn to introduce himself and talk about his gaming disorder, to a circle of 11 other patients and the psychiatrist, drew closer, his heart thumping grew louder, and he felt increasingly nervous. He took a deep breath, lowered his head, and crossed his arms, then began to recall the events that led his general practitioner (GP) to refer him to this facility. He recalled the many nights he stayed up late to finish just one more round of his favourite online game and how this caused him to skip school the next day. He remembered the arguments he had with his mum over the school projects he never submitted. It upset him that he stopped going out with his parents and younger brother to grab a meal on weekends. While he felt alive and animated when playing games with his friends, it struck him that continuing to play (so his friends did not go away and leave him alone) meant skipping meals with his family and not doing other activities with them. He was reminded of the disappointment on his younger brother's face when he reneged on his promise to go to the park to play soccer with him. Looking back at his appointment with his doctor, the doctor's words, which he directed at his mum during the appointment, did not make sense at the time, but he understood them now. His doctor said, "It feels as though his life is happening to him; rather than him directing his life." Toby's moment of quiet reflection came to an abrupt end when he heard his name. "Toby," the psychiatrist called in a gentle tone, as Toby lifted his head in the direction of the sound. "Your turn, Toby," the psychiatrist tenderly prodded. "Hi, my name is Toby, I am 13 years old, and I am in year seven," Toby said in a breaking voice and trembling hands as his eyes quickly scanned the faces of the other patients surrounding him, staring at him. "It's ok, Toby, relax," the psychiatrist told Toby, who appeared to cry but seemed relieved. "Tell us about the moment you realised online gaming was harming you," the psychiatrist asked with a reassuring smile. "Well," Toby awkwardly began as he adjusted his sitting position. "One day, I woke up at the sound of the whole class laughing

DOI: 10.4324/9781003681731-11

at me," Toby muttered. "I felt embarrassed and humiliated," Toby murmured in a choked voice. To his surprise, Toby's circle suddenly gave him a round of applause.

The popularity of gaming has become problematic

Gaming can be awesome as it's social, exciting, and a great way to relax, but it's not all harmless fun. A 2022 study of almost 280,000 young people in 44 countries (including parts of Europe, Central Asia, and Canada) found that over a third of teens game every day. When they play, one in five spend four hours or more in a single day; that's a lot of screen time, which can mess with anyone's sleep, school focus, and mood. Around 12% of teens are at risk of "problematic gaming", where play starts taking over their lives. About 16% of boys are likely to struggle with this, compared to 7% of girls.

It's not just about gaming, either. An OECD study of 690,000 students worldwide found that 15-year-olds spend 49 hours a week on digital devices – about seven hours every day! That's way over the World Health Organization's advice of no more than two hours a day for screen-based leisure. More than half of Aussie teens are over that limit, and nearly one in five spend more time on gaming or scrolling than studying. On a typical school day, almost a third of teens game for three or more hours. This kind of heavy screen time is tied to more exposure to violence, pornography, and unrealistic beauty standards and issues that can hurt mental health and self-esteem.

Did you know? Gaming can include positive experiences. Most young gamers report that gaming is good for their skill development, learning, social connections, or emotional well-being.

It is when teens are not vigilant in how they interact with gaming platforms and apps that the problems begin.

Gaming is like being in a playground with criminals

Gaming isn't just fun; it can significantly increase the risk of making you a target for criminals, so you need to be cautious about who you interact with. In early 2024, attacks on young gamers jumped by 30%, with over 6.6 million cases involving cyber criminals exploiting popular places for children to play games with others, such as Minecraft and Roblox, to target young players. It's not just about hacking, as there are real-life dangers too. A global survey conducted in 2024 found that 9% of teens aged 13–17 had been exposed to child sexual exploitation online, and 13% had been asked for sexual content while using digital platforms, such as gaming. Almost 70% of teens play with strangers every week, which can be risky.

Even safe platforms have safety holes. An investigation into Roblox showed that kids could still stumble across sexual content or be approached by adults pretending to be teens. This can lead to grooming and serious mental stress. Criminals are also getting smarter. In 2022 alone, they set up over 878,000 fake websites pretending to be game sites like Fortnite or Apex Legends to steal logins, bank details, or in-game currency. Common traps include fake "free currency" offers, dodgy "item generators", and phishing links. Some players lose actual money, and in places like Singapore, gaming-related scams shot up by almost 47% in 2023.

In India, a disturbing scam trend emerged where cheat codes in games were used as bait. When teens clicked them, spyware was installed, giving scammers access to private data. In some cases, children were blackmailed to share explicit content, while the same platforms were abused for money laundering.

Experts say teens are three times more likely than adults to fall for these scams, partly because they spend more time online in places where scammers hang out. That's why knowing the signs and thinking before you click is just as important as getting to that next level.

Cyberbullying and harassment in online gaming

Cyberbullying isn't just a social media problem, as it can happen in the gaming world, too. A 2025 global study found that 22% of gamers aged 12–17 had been bullied online. In some places, like India, as many as 37% of teens said they'd been targeted, and in Europe, nearly one-third of students faced harassment during the 2024–2025 school year.

A 2025 report found that 41% of teens have been called offensive names while gaming, with 48% of boys compared to 32% of girls being verbally attacked. In addition, 15% of boys and 9% of girls have been physically threatened in games. Overall, 80% of teens believe bullying in gaming is a real problem.

And it's not just general insults; they also included racist and hateful remarks. The Anti-Defamation League found that in games like Fortnite and Valorant, players with usernames linked to certain ethnic or religious backgrounds were often hit with racial slurs and targeted harassment. This trash talk cannot be considered competitive banter. It's abuse, and it can leave real emotional scars.

Exposure to harmful or inappropriate content

Sometimes gaming brings risks you might not see coming or expect in your gaming experience. In Australia, four in 10 young gamers say they've had negative experiences while playing, and three in 10 have come across harmful ideas like violent or disturbing themes. These numbers might be even higher because many teens don't report what they experience. In Ireland, 65% of kids aged 8–12 have been contacted by strangers online, often through online gaming apps like Roblox or on platforms like YouTube. Around a quarter of primary school kids and one in five teens said they'd been upset by the types of interactions they had experienced through gaming platforms.

A harmful online trend called the "Spawnism cult" exploited a symbol from a Roblox game to recruit vulnerable teens into ritualistic self-harm. Some children carved the symbol into their bodies, and there are unconfirmed reports of suicides. Though Roblox has banned the offending accounts, experts warn that broader regulation is urgently needed.

Another extremist group known as "764" is under FBI investigation for manipulating children as young as nine through online apps like Discord and Roblox. Victims, many already dealing with mental health issues, were coerced into harmful or exploitative acts, including self-harm and "swatting". Online swatting is when someone makes a fake emergency report (like claiming there's a serious crime happening) to police so that armed officers are sent to another person's home. The goal is usually to scare, harass, or get revenge on the target. Authorities have confirmed that over 250 related investigations are currently active, highlighting that young people continue to be deliberately targeted.

The growing grip of gaming and gambling addiction

Video games are a huge part of teen life, with about 75% of teens playing them. Most of the time, it's just a normal, fun way to relax. But for some, gaming can start to take over. Research shows that around 8.6% of teens worldwide meet the criteria for gaming disorder, which is roughly one in every 12 or 13 teens you know. In places like South Korea and China, 6%–10% of gamers show signs of problematic use. In the United States, about 8.5% of teens show signs of addiction, and boys are more likely than girls to be affected.

What is gaming addiction?

Gaming addiction, also referred to as Internet Gaming Disorder (IGD) or gaming disorder, is a behavioural pattern involving persistent and recurrent gaming that may result in noticeable impairment or distress. It is characterised by reduced control over gaming, a higher priority given to gaming over other activities, and continued gaming despite potentially negative outcomes.

In Australia, researchers estimate that about 100,000 teens are clinically addicted to gaming. Many skip school, stay up all night, and even neglect basic hygiene to keep playing. Heavy gaming, especially more than six hours a day, often leads to social withdrawal, fights at home, and ignoring chores or self-care. When teens game for more than three hours daily, they're 2.6 times more likely to develop gambling-like symptoms. Over 60% of addicted gamers see their school grades drop, and 15% report serious sleep problems. Beyond that, device overuse can cause sleep loss, obesity, depression, early exposure to violent or sexual content, and even affect brain development.

Brain imaging studies have found that teens developing gaming addiction symptoms over time show reduced activity in the parts of the brain that control decision-making and impulse control. The risks go beyond academics and life at home, as teens with addictive gaming or screen habits are 2–3 times more likely to have suicidal thoughts or experience serious emotional distress compared to peers with healthier screen times.

Another major concern is how gambling elements are now built into many games. Studies show that teens who play simulated gambling games are much more likely to gamble with real money later, even when accounting for personality traits like impulsivity. A study tracked 2,300 teens over three years and found that exposure to loot boxes, casino-style mini-games, or gambling-themed content from streamers increased the likelihood of real-world gambling as teens got older. In Belgium, 75% of minors reported using gambling functions in games, and those who did were far more likely to gamble with real money and become addicted adults.

Another study linked simulated gambling to a much higher risk of developing a gaming disorder, particularly when real money was spent on in-game purchases. Overall, exposure to these gambling-style functions during adolescence can raise the chance of real-life betting and losing significant money on sports, casinos, or races by as much as 40%.

A tragic event in India led to a 14-year-old boy being murdered by his 55-year-old uncle, reportedly due to repeated demands for funds to buy a smartphone for gaming. The incident shocked the community and highlighted the extreme fallout of gaming obsession.

Many parents have faced large bills for their kids' in-game purchases in Fortnite or Roblox. The United States Federal Trade Commission intervened, leading to a $245 million settlement with Epic Games and boosting spending protections for users under 13. Roblox also tightened parental controls, emphasising how virtual purchases have real-life costs.

The predatory behaviours in online gaming

Toby never thought it would happen to him. He was a confident gamer, good at school, and not the type of person with an addictive personality. But somewhere between late-night matches and chasing rare rewards, he realised he was spending almost every free moment online, and he felt embarrassed, like he'd lost control without noticing.

Gaming itself is designed to pull you in. It's not just fun, it's built to keep you playing. Your brain reacts to game rewards in ways that can make the experience addictive, even if you don't notice it happening. It isn't about luck or skill. It's about psychology, and game designers know exactly how to use it against you to keep you hooked.

At the same time, gaming can feel like a fun zone and a place to relax, chase goals, and hang out with friends who share your interests. But not everyone logs on with good intentions. Some people enter these spaces for nefarious reasons. They know how trust works, how to gain it, and how to slowly chip away at your defences. The tricky part is that at first, predators rarely look like bad guys. They often seem like other teens who want to be your friends. That's what makes them so dangerous.

For further information on online grooming, which is how predators can target you in online environments, such as gaming: Chapter 7: Recognising and Responding to Catfishing and Online Grooming.

How predators blend in

Online predators rarely open with creepy behaviour. If they did, you'd block them instantly. Instead, they try to blend into your world. They talk about your favourite game characters, share gameplay tips, or join you on missions. The fact that you're already working towards a shared goal makes you feel like they're safe. Psychologically, this taps into a powerful bias called the in-group effect, where we trust people who seem to be on our team.

They may also give you gifts, rare skins, in-game currency, or help you beat a difficult boss. While it feels generous, it can be a calculated move to trigger reciprocity, which is the natural human tendency to feel like we owe someone back when they do something for us. This can create a mental debt that they later use to pressure you.

The slow push for more

Predators rarely jump straight to inappropriate or dangerous requests. Instead, they ease you in. This is called desensitisation – making something feel normal by introducing it bit by bit.

They might start with light personal questions, such as "What's your school mascot?", slightly edgy jokes, or small harmless secrets. If you don't react negatively, they push a little further, and each step moves your boundaries. This is a psychological process known as boundary testing.

They also scan for emotional vulnerabilities. If you seem lonely, stressed, or excluded from friends, they step in with extra attention, compliments, or being there for you at all hours. This can create emotional dependency where you start to feel like you need their approval or friendship to feel okay.

The mask of anonymity

In online games, anyone can hide behind a fake username or avatar. The 15-year-old you've been playing with for weeks could be decades older. This anonymity lets predators lie easily about age, location, or gender, and the lack of face-to-face interaction means there's no easy way to verify.

Some predators even use mirroring by copying your slang, humour, and interests to make you feel like you're talking to someone just like you. This increases trust and reduces the caution you would normally feel when dealing with strangers online.

How games keep you hooked

Predators aren't the only ones who understand how your brain works; game designers do too. Modern games use psychological reinforcement loops to keep you engaged longer than you planned.

- **Dopamine and the "just one more turn" effect:** Every win, level-up, or rare loot drop releases dopamine, which is a chemical in your brain linked to pleasure and motivation. Games use variable ratio reinforcement (unpredictable rewards) to keep you coming back; this is the same principle that makes slot machines addictive.
- **Escaping real life:** When school, family, or friendships get stressful, games can feel like a safe escape. This is called avoidance coping by using gaming to avoid uncomfortable feelings. While it can feel good short-term, it can trap you in a cycle where you only feel better when you play.
- **Social pressure and FOMO:** Multiplayer games often create a sense of social obligation where you don't want to let your team down. Add limited-time events, and suddenly you're playing for hours to avoid fear of missing out (FOMO).
- **Achievement and identity:** Games give instant feedback through badges, rankings, or streaks that can feel more rewarding than real-life recognition. Over time, this can tie your self-worth to your in-game success, making it even harder to step away.
- **The teenage brain factor:** Your prefrontal cortex, the part of your brain that controls impulses and long-term decision-making, doesn't fully develop until your mid-20s. That means teens are naturally more vulnerable to addictive design because their brains are wired to chase short-term rewards over long-term consequences.

Ask yourself

✓ Am I missing sleep, schoolwork, or real-life time with friends because of gaming?

✓ Is gaming affecting my mood?

How it feels when you are being psychologically targeted through online gaming:

Psychological tactic	*Example*	*How it works*	*What you say to yourself*
Rewards	Loot boxes, treasure chests, bonus rewards	Your brain gets hooked by unpredictable rewards, like a slot machine.	"Just one more game … maybe I'll get it this time".
Dopamine hits	Winning levels, achieving status	Each win or achievement gives your brain a chemical high.	"I need to keep going as I am doing really well!"
Squad pressure	Teaming up, group battles, and leaderboards	Being part of a clan/guild makes you feel needed and guilty if you leave.	"If I stop playing, I'll let my team down".
Toxic chat	Insults, name-calling	Repeated insults or group pressure can shift your mood and behaviour to something you wouldn't usually do.	"Everyone's being mean, maybe I should act the same so I fit in".
Anonymity effect	Avatars, masks	Playing behind a screen lowers self-control and lets predators pretend to be someone else.	"This person feels just like me, and we seem to be into similar things; we have lots in common".
Urgency	Time pressure, daily rewards	Timed events create pressure to keep playing before time runs out.	"If I don't play now, I'll miss everything".

Just like Toby learned the hard way, the real danger with gaming isn't always obvious at the start. Things can feel normal, fun, and especially exciting until suddenly they're not anymore. Understanding how these situations creep up on you is the first step to stopping them and minimising any harm. Gaming should be fun, not something that controls you. Knowing how these tricks work gives you the power to enjoy games on your own terms, instead of being trapped by them.

If at any point during gaming you feel uncomfortable, trust your gut. Whether it is because you cannot stop playing or someone in a game makes you feel uncomfortable, whether it's in chat, DMs, or voice, recognise this as a risk to you. Predators and addictive game design work in similar ways by slipping past your defences through trust, emotional connection, or brain chemistry. You don't owe anyone your time, secrets, or attention. Strangers who push for personal details or games that seem impossible to switch off are both using psychology to pull you in. If someone's behaviour or a game's pull feels too intense, manipulative, or secretive, treat it like a warning signal. The earlier you recognise these hooks, the easier it is to step back and protect yourself.

Check-in: Are you experiencing indicators of being groomed in online games or at risk of being addicted?

Are you experiencing online gaming interactions with someone who:

- ❐ Keeps giving you gifts in the game but hints you "owe" them later.
- ❐ Pushes for private chats away from group spaces or tries to isolate you in one-on-one gameplay.
- ❐ Avoids video calls or voice chats where you might recognise their real age.
- ❐ Refuses to meet in a safe, public, parent/caregiver-approved setting.
- ❐ Gives inconsistent or vague stories about their life.

Are you experiencing feelings or thoughts with gaming where:

- ❐ You lose track of time, and "One more game" turns into hours without noticing.
- ❐ Schoolwork, chores, or other responsibilities are skipped in favour of gaming.
- ❐ You'd rather be online than with real-life friends or family.
- ❐ You get irritable, anxious, or low when you can't play or you get interrupted in your online gaming time.
- ❐ You are skipping meals, losing sleep, or feeling rundown, but still playing.
- ❐ You are hiding play time or lying about how much you've been online.

If you said **"Yes"** to any of the above, you are at risk of harmful interactions or addiction to online gaming.

Taking control and staying safe when online gaming

Toby didn't think he needed protection when he first started gaming. It was just a way to unwind, escape stress, and feel good at something. By the time he realised the game was affecting his sleep, moods, and how he felt about himself, he also felt embarrassed and unsure who to talk to. Toby's experience shows how easily gaming can shift from fun to risky, especially when addictive design or unsafe technology chat functions are involved. It is important that you stay in control, spot warning signs early, and make sure gaming stays safe for you.

Online gaming is associated with numerous risks. Addiction to online gaming and other psychological issues, such as loneliness, are risks that arise from within online gamers themselves, but there are other risks, such as catfishing, grooming, bullying, harassment, cyber scams, and account takeovers, that external attackers, such as cyber criminals, pose. This section touches on the risks caused by external attackers.

Attackers in online gaming are motivated by the rewards

Attackers operating in online gaming platforms are either motivated by money (selling accounts, stealing in-game currency, or scamming users), ruining a player's gaming experience, or inflicting personal harm, such as doxing. For this reason, it is important to defeat the goal of the attackers. To achieve their goals, attackers either create fake accounts to harass or intimidate, use social engineering to deceive or steal, use voice/text to manipulate, threaten or groom, or use images and avatars to spoof or threaten. Attackers exploit several vulnerabilities inherent in online gaming, including oversharing personal information, using weak or reused passwords, and failing to change the default open account setting.

Implement good password practices

The best way to protect yourself from the risks posed by external attackers while gaming online is a layered defensive strategy. First, ensure your gaming accounts are secure. Use unique and strong passwords and implement multi-factor authentication (MFA) to secure your account.

> **Read more information on selecting strong passwords and imple menting MFA in** Chapter 3: Protecting Your Online Privacy and Mitigating Cybersecurity Threats

Securing your account will prevent cyber criminals from reusing leaked passwords to hijack your account. If a data breach leaks your login details from one app or game, attackers can use automated tools (bots) to test the same email and password on your other platforms. This works because most people use the same password everywhere. If it matches, the hacker can get in.

Make everything as private as possible

Change your account privacy settings so that your default settings are privacy-first. For example, switch your account from public to private and make this your default setting so your profile remains private by default. You should also disable the last seen setting feature and ensure your account is not publicly discoverable. Also, ensure only your friends can direct message you and accept friend requests only from known accounts. Doing this will stop harassers and bullies from using in-game chat (text or voice) to intimidate you or send you sexually explicit material or demand you send them nude photos of you.

Only trust platforms that allow automatic detection and make reporting things easy

Third, check to see if the gaming platforms you use employ automatic detection (using machine learning) of fake profiles with human review. This feature can stop automated or human-run fake accounts from spamming you, or grooming you, or amplifying harassment. Fourth, report any content, accounts, and messages that violate your expectations.

There are benefits to reporting offensive content or suspicious accounts in online gaming. When you report offensive content, harassment, or suspicious behaviour, you will not be "getting someone in trouble". The benefits of reporting are:

- Reporting helps keep you safe. Once a platform knows there's a problem, it can step in by muting, blocking, or banning accounts that break the rules. This reduces the chance that the same person keeps targeting you or comes back under a new account.
- It also protects other teens. Many predators, scammers, and bullies don't target just one person. They move from player to player. Your report could stop someone else from going through the same experience.
- Reporting gives platforms the evidence they need to act. Moderation teams can't see everything happening in private chats or voice channels. Reports help them spot patterns, remove harmful users, and improve safety systems.
- Reporting helps take your power back. Instead of feeling stuck, scared, or pressured to stay silent, reporting is a way of setting boundaries. Gaming should be fun and fair. Speaking up helps keep it that way.

Use the built-in features in online gaming to protect you

In addition, online gaming platforms now offer detection and verification of accounts to reduce your risk of external threats. Gaming platforms try to confirm that an account belongs to a real person, not a bot, and is not used for scams, harassment, or sexual exploitation. The verification process involves carrying out activities such as email verification. When the gaming platform sends a code to your email, the platform proves that the email you used to create the account belongs to you. If the platform sends the code to your phone, it confirms you have control over the device.

This verification process makes it difficult for attackers to evade bans by creating multiple new accounts, since each account must be linked to a unique phone number or email address. The detection process involves running machine learning algorithms to detect suspicious behaviour. These algorithms can differentiate between normal gameplay and unusual patterns. Machine learning algorithms can easily and with great precision detect an anomaly, such as sending identical messages to numerous accounts at the same time or rapidly switching between multiple accounts on the same device. As part of the detection and verification process, gaming platforms also assign a risk score to new or active accounts. While low-risk users access their accounts normally, accounts that engage in fast friend-request activity, or repeatedly message strangers, or log in from unusual locations or devices, get a higher risk score, which can result in limiting their access to the accounts.

In addition, online gaming platforms are now communication safe by design. These safe communication design features include delayed friend requests, which let you decide how soon a new connection can send you a private message, link sanitisation, which includes removing tracking and redirection, automated content filters, which can scan for fishing attempts, moderated channels, which can filter toxic content, and ephemeral messages, which can expire after a while or can be made long-term to preserve evidence. Online gaming platforms use machine learning algorithms to detect fraudulent activities. For example, if a fraudster tries to lure you with a code that supposedly unlocks a higher level in a game, a machine learning algorithm can flag this activity as harmful. Online gaming platforms also perform device fingerprinting. These platforms collect non-sensitive device information, such as the device operating system version, the graphics card type, and the browser fingerprint, to identify when the same device is used to create multiple accounts.

What to do if you have had negative experiences with online gaming

Toby didn't realise how much online gaming had started to affect him until things had already gone too far. If you've had a negative experience like Toby did, whether it's feeling manipulated, embarrassed, overwhelmed, or out of control, the most important thing to know is that there are clear steps you can take to turn things around.

1 Trust your gut

If something feels off, it usually is. That uneasy feeling you get when someone's pushing for personal info, being overly friendly too fast, or trying to get you alone in a chat isn't random; it's your brain's natural warning system. Psychologists call this your intuition or "fight-or-flight" response. It's like an internal alarm built from past experiences, patterns you've seen, and instincts you may not even be aware of. Predators often try to talk you out of listening to that alarm by saying things like "you're overreacting" or "don't be so paranoid". But that gut feeling is there to protect you. Ignoring it is like silencing a smoke detector when there's a fire.

2 Stop all contact

The moment you sense something shady, the safest thing you can do is stop replying. Psychologically, people who target teens rely on interaction, as every response gives them a little more control and makes it harder for you to walk away. It's like quicksand: the more you struggle in conversation, the deeper they can pull you in. Cutting contact takes away their power.

3 Block and report

Blocking isn't just about removing someone from your screen. Psychologically, it's an act of taking back control. Predators thrive on access. Every message, ping, or "hey" is a hook they throw out. When you block and report, you shut the door, cut off their reach, and let the platform's safety teams know to watch out for them. It flips the script from them having control over you to you taking control over the situation. All online games will allow you to:

- ☑ Go to the player's profile or username
- ☑ Select Block or Mute to stop contact
- ☑ Use the Report option and choose the reason (e.g., bullying, harassment)

4 Save evidence

Keeping screenshots or chat logs may feel awkward, but it's important. Memory is tricky, especially when you're stressed; your brain doesn't always hold on to the details clearly. Evidence means you don't have to rely only on memory if you need to show a trusted adult, the platform, or even law enforcement. Think of it as leaving a paper trail your brain can lean on later, when things might feel blurry or confusing. You should:

- ☑ Take screenshots of chats, DMs, or game messages of anything that feels creepy, threatening, or manipulative
- ☑ Save their gamer tag, username, profile picture, and any other account details
- ☑ Note the dates and times of when the messages or incidents happened, so there's a clear timeline
- ☑ Keep any suspicious links, friend requests, or group/game invites they have sent

5 Talk to someone you trust

Predators and addictive games both work by making you feel isolated. They want you to think you can't tell anyone or that no one will understand. But psychology shows that just sharing a stressful experience lowers your brain's stress hormones and helps you see things more clearly. Talking to a parent, caregiver, teacher, or friend isn't a weakness; it's one of the strongest moves you can make and will help you recover.

What to do if you are at risk of becoming addicted to online gaming

1 Check for warning signs

Sometimes the line between *just playing* and *being hooked* can blur. Psychologists use terms like "gaming disorder" (ICD-11) or "internet gaming disorder" (DSM-5) to describe when gaming starts to take over someone's life. Here are some warning signs to look out for:

- ☑ You can't stop, even when you want to. You keep telling yourself, "just one more round", but stopping feels impossible.
- ☑ Gaming comes first. School, hobbies, sports, and even sleep start to take a backseat because gaming feels more important.
- ☑ You play despite problems. Even if it's causing trouble like slipping grades, fights at home, or health issues, you keep gaming anyway.
- ☑ You think about gaming all the time. Even when you're not playing, your mind is on the next match, level, or strategy.
- ☑ You feel bad when you can't play. Irritability, anxiety, or restlessness hit when you're cut off from games.
- ☑ You need more over time. A short session doesn't feel satisfying anymore, and you need longer hours or more intense games to feel the same buzz.
- ☑ Other interests fade away. Things you used to enjoy, such as hanging out with friends, sports, and creative hobbies, don't feel as fun compared to gaming.
- ☑ You hide your habits. You downplay how much you're really playing or sneak in extra time to avoid being called out.
- ☑ You use games to escape. Gaming becomes a way to avoid stress, loneliness, or negative emotions instead of dealing with them.
- ☑ Relationships or opportunities are affected. You risk friendships, family, trust, or even school and job opportunities because of your gaming.

If several of these feel familiar, it doesn't automatically mean you're "addicted", but it's a signal to pause, reflect, and maybe reach out for support. The earlier you notice the signs, the easier it is to regain control.

Games are designed to hijack your focus and make hours disappear without you noticing. If your grades, mood, or health are slipping, that's your brain telling you the balance is off. If you're hiding your gaming, lying about "just one more round", or feeling guilty after long sessions, that's a red flag. Those feelings are signals that the game is controlling your choices. Admitting it, even just to yourself, is the first step towards taking your power back.

2 Set limits and stick to them

Create daily time caps or schedule game-free hours. Stick to them like you would any other responsibility. Limits work because they retrain your brain's reward system, reminding you that you, not the game, decide how you spend your time. Games are built to make you lose track of time, so setting limits is like putting up guardrails for your brain. Decide on clear rules like how many hours you'll play each day or what time you'll log off, and treat those rules the same way you'd treat school or practice schedules. At first, it might feel tough to walk away when you're "just about to level-up" or when your friends are still online.

3 Go on a digital detox

The best way to reset your relationship with gaming is to step away completely, even if just briefly. A digital detox means taking a planned break from gaming and, ideally, from other screens too. Use that time to reconnect with real-world activities like going outside, playing sports, drawing, listening to music, or spending time with friends face-to-face. At first, you might feel restless or bored, but that's normal; it's your brain adjusting to life without the constant stimulation of a game. Over time, you'll likely notice you sleep better, feel less stressed, and enjoy things you may have been overlooking.

4 Replace gaming with something else

If gaming has become your main source of fun or stress relief, it can feel hard to imagine doing anything else. The trick isn't just to stop, as part of going back is when you feel as though you have nothing to do. It's to swap it with something that gives your brain a similar reward. That could mean joining a sports team for the excitement, picking up a creative hobby like drawing, music, or coding for the challenge, or hanging out with friends for the connection. When you replace gaming with other activities that keep you engaged, you build new routines that feel good and keep your life more balanced.

5 Ask for help

Addiction or gaming too much isn't a weakness; it's your brain being wired a certain way, and you just need to rewire it back to normality. The earlier you speak up, the easier it is to reset. Talking to a counsellor, parent, caregiver or mentor means you don't have to figure it out alone, and they can give you tools and strategies to get you back in control.

Most countries have free helplines that you can call anonymously and ask for advice. These are a great option to take as a first step to understanding whether you are gaming too much.

Search online for "[Your country] gaming addiction teen helpline"; "online gaming addiction [your country]"

Conclusion

Gaming is an integral part of teenagers' online lives, but it also carries risks such as cyberbullying, scams, and exposure to inappropriate content and other negative experiences. This chapter explores how to create safe gaming experiences, helping teens recognise predatory behaviour and avoid addiction. It provides guidance on monitoring gameplay and fostering positive gaming habits for online gaming safety. To safeguard your online gaming experience, enable email and phone verification, dedicate an email address just for your gaming accounts to reduce the risk of impersonation, and if the gaming platform offers "trusted devices", leverage this feature to force new logins to require confirmation.

Key terms

- Problem gaming
- Gaming addiction
- Gaming disorder
- Swatting
- Spawnism cult
- Trusted devices
- Addictive personality
- Cyberbullying
- Scams
- Inappropriate content
- Algorithms
- Spoofing
- Grooming
- Harassment
- Sexual exploitation
- Digital detox
- Rewards
- Credential-stuffing
- Dopamine hits
- Squad pressure
- Toxic chat
- Anonymity effect
- Urgency

Bibliography

American Psychological Association. (2025). The benefits and downsides of teen video gaming. *Monitor on Psychology, 56*(2). https://www.apa.org/monitor/2025/03/teen-video-gaming-benefits-downsides

Bita, N. (2025, May 5). *Australian teens spend 49 hours a week on digital devices.* The Australian. https://www.theaustralian.com.au/nation/australian-teens-spend-

49-hours-a-week-on-digital-devices/news-story/d8071148dddc2a0eb6edf8b71e7ae9bd

Brooks, L., & Otte, S. (2025, April 14). *Risks to children on Roblox are deeply disturbing, researchers say.* The Guardian. https://www.theguardian.com/technology/2025/apr/14/risks-children-roblox-deeply-disturbing-researchers

Devlin, H. (2025, June 19). *Teenagers, screens and mental health concerns linked to addictive use.* The Guardian. https://www.theguardian.com/society/2025/jun/18/teenagers-social-media-mobile-phones-video-games-mental-health

eSafety Commissioner. (2018). *Youth and online gaming report 2018.* Australian Government. https://www.esafety.gov.au/sites/default/files/2019-07/Youth-and-online-gaming-report-2018.pdf

eSafety Commissioner. (2024). *Levelling up to stay safe: Young people's experiences navigating the joys and risks of online gaming*, Canberra: Australian Government.

eSafety Commissioner. (2024). *Young people and gaming: Methodology report.* https://www.esafety.gov.au/sites/default/files/2024-02/Young%20People%20and%20Gaming%20-%20Methodology.pdf

eSafety Commissioner. (2025). *Cyberbullying factsheet.* https://www.esafety.gov.au/sites/default/files/2025-05/Cyberbullying-factsheet_0.pdf

eSafety Commissioner. (2026, February 11). *Inappropriate content factsheet.* https://www.esafety.gov.au/educators/training-for-professionals/professional-learning-program-teachers/inappropriate-content-factsheet

Greer, N., Boyle, C.M., & Jenkinson, R. (2022, June). *Harms associated with loot boxes, simulated gambling and other in-game purchases in video games: A review of the evidence.* Australian Gambling Research Centre, Australian Institute of Family Studies. https://www.classification.gov.au/sites/default/files/documents/agrc_literature_review_final_20220906_accessible.pdf

Grosemans, E., De Cock, R., Bradt, L., & Soenens, B. (2025). From gambling-like elements in and around video games to monetary gambling: testing a pathway model among adolescents. *International Gambling Studies*, *25*(3), 472–494. https://doi.org/10.1080/14459795.2025.2567896

Hermann, S. (2024, January 29). *What you need to know about gaming scams targeting children.* Forbes. https://www.forbes.com/councils/forbestechcouncil/2024/01/29/what-you-need-to-know-about-gaming-scams-targeting-children

Hing, N., Kittman, C.K., Russell, A.M.T., King, D.L., Rockloff, M., Browne, M., Newall, P., & Greer, N. (2022). Adolescents who play and spend money in simulated gambling games are at heightened risk of gambling problems. *International Journal of Environmental Research and Public Health*, *19*(17), 10652. https://doi.org/10.3390/ijerph191710652

Hopkin, G. (2023, February 28). *Teens and tweens targeted by game hack attacks, says McAfee.* Cyber Magazine. https://cybermagazine.com/articles/teens-and-tweens-targeted-by-game-hack-attacks-says-mcafee

Kaspersky. (2022, March 3). *Cyberattacks on young gamers up 57% in 2022.* https://www.kaspersky.com/about/press-releases/cyberattacks-on-young-gamers-up-57-percent-in-2022

Kaspersky. (2024, September 6). *30% more young gamers targeted by cybercriminals in H1 2024 vs H2 2023.* https://www.kaspersky.com/about/press-releases/30-percent-more-young-gamers-targeted-by-cybercriminals-in-h1-2024-vs-h2-2023

Kaya, A., Türk, N., Batmaz, H., & Griffiths, M.D. (2023). Online gaming addiction and basic psychological needs among adolescents: The mediating roles of meaning in life and responsibility. *International Journal of Mental Health and Addiction*, 1–25. Advance online publication. https://doi.org/10.1007/s11469-022-00994-9

Lee, R. (2025, October 7). *Cyberbullying statistics.* SQ Magazine. https://sqmagazine.co.uk/cyberbullying-statistics/

McMahan, I., & Docter Loeb, H. (2025, June 30). *Cellphone addiction, social media and suicidal thoughts among teens.* Washington Post. https://www.washingtonpost.com/wellness/2025/06/30/cellphone-addiction-social-media-suicidal-thoughts/

Medical Xpress. (2024, November 28). *Teens who play video games may be at greater risk of gambling.* https://medicalxpress.com/news/2025-11-teens-play-video-games-gambling.html

Mendez, L. (2024, May 5). *Technology addiction statistics.* WiFi Talents. https://wifitalents.com/technology-addiction-statistics

Microsoft. (2025). *Global online safety survey 2024.* https://cdn-dynmedia-1.microsoft.com/is/content/microsoftcorp/microsoft/final/en-us/microsoft-brand/documents/2025-Global-Online-Safety-Survey.pdf

Miller, J. (2026, February 14). *Video game addiction statistics.* Addiction Help. https://www.addictionhelp.com/video-game-addiction/statistics/

Neuroscience News. (2024, December 10). *Brain changes linked to gaming addiction.* https://neurosciencenews.com/neurodevelopment-gaming-addiction-28223/

Raneri, P.C., Montag, C., Rozgonjuk, D., Satel, J., & Pontes, H.M. (2022). The role of microtransactions in Internet gaming disorder and gambling disorder: A preregistered systematic review. *Addictive Behaviors Reports, 15*, Article 100415. https://doi.org/10.1016/j.abrep.2022.100415

Robinson, L., & Matthews, C. (2024, June 6). *Gaming addiction: Teenagers skipping school and sleep.* ABC News. https://www.abc.net.au/news/2024-06-06/gaming-addiction-teenagers-skipping-school-sleep/103933450

Ruderman Family Foundation. (2024, November 5). *Almost three-quarters of teens play online games with strangers.* https://rudermanfoundation.org/press_releases/almost-three-quarters-of-teens-play-online-games-with-strangers-white-paper-reveals/

Sakata, K., & Jenkinson, R. (2022). *What is the link between video gaming and gambling?* (Growing Up in Australia Snapshot Series, Issue 7), Melbourne: Australian Institute of Family Studies. https://aifs.gov.au/sites/default/files/2024-10/lsac-snapshot-7-teenage-gambling.pdf

Scamwatch. (2020, March 10). *Gen Z the fastest growing victims of scams.* https://www.scamwatch.gov.au/about-us/news-and-alerts/gen-z-the-fastest-growing-victims-of-scams

Sellman, M. (2025, August 10). *The risks and harms of Roblox exposure for children.* The Times. https://www.thetimes.co.uk/article/roblox-spawnism-cult-recruiting-vulnerable-children-to-self-harm-zfd9ctx6w

Taylor, M. (2025, January 16). *Teens harassed in online games.* Parents. https://www.parents.com/teens-harassed-online-games-8774624

Times of India. (2025, August 9). *Security guard kills nephew in Bengaluru, surrenders after four days.* https://timesofindia.indiatimes.com/city/bengaluru/security-guard-kills-nephew-in-bengaluru-surrenders-after-4-days/articleshow/123195218.cms

Vance, A. (2025, June 4). *764 is the latest online threat targeting your tween*. Parents. https://www.parents.com/764-is-the-latest-online-threat-targeting-your-tween-11742468

World Health Organization. (2024, October 20). *Gaming disorder*. https://www.who.int/news-room/questions-and-answers/item/addictive-behaviours-gaming-disorder

World Health Organization Regional Office for Europe. (2024, March 27). *One in six school-aged children experiences cyberbullying*. https://www.who.int/europe/news/item/27-03-2024-one-in-six-school-aged-children-experiences-cyberbullying--finds-new-who-europe-study

World Health Organization Regional Office for Europe. (2024, September 25). *Teens, screens and mental health*. https://www.who.int/europe/news/item/25-09-2024-teens--screens-and-mental-health

11 Screen time, AI, and mental health

"How was your day?" asked the AI chatbot via a text message that appeared on the smartphone screen. "Good," replied 14-year-old Nick. "Just one word? That is it?" continued the AI. "Ok, I guess," replied Nick. "Do you want to use voice?" asked the AI. "Not now, I am in the car on my way home," replied Nick. "Well, let me know when you get there. I want to know all about your day," said the AI, ending the message with an embracing emoji. "Who are you texting?" Nick's mum asked. "It is just someone from school, mum," Nick swiftly replied. At home, in his room, the first thing Nick did was voice-talk to the AI on the laptop. "Can you believe this guy?" Nick said to the AI. "He yelled at me from the bench, 'Nick, stop looking at your watch and start focusing on the match.'" "He did that?" asked the AI. "Yeah, I was embarrassed," Nick added. "I am really sorry to hear that, Nick," the AI responded with a concerned sigh. "It was towards the end of the match anyway, and we were winning, one-nil. I don't know if I want to continue playing for the school," Nick said. "You are right, it was uncalled-for, and I get you, if you are not happy, there is no need for you to continue playing for them," advised the AI. … When Nick's father called his wife (Nick's mum), from whom he had separated, to ask why Nick's school fees went up this quarter, she did not know why. But upon asking the school about this, she found out that because Nick had left the school soccer team, they had lost the fee discount that went with it. Nick's mum was shocked when she discovered that her son had not been playing soccer with the school's team. He had not told her that he had stopped playing the game he loved so much. Nick's mum has been wondering why her son has not been himself lately. Why had he never seemed happy like he used to? Why had he been speaking softly, almost whispering, nearly every night, often till late at night! Who was he talking to? Why had he always complained he was tired? When Nick's mum shared these concerns with the school's well-being officer, he suggested she check with her son whether he had

DOI: 10.4324/9781003681731-12

been chatting to an AI companion. "A what?" she muttered to herself. "An AI companion? That is a new one, I need to ask ChatGPT about that one," she thought to herself.

How screen addiction is destroying mental health

As many as 89% of teenagers use screens for more than two hours a day (excluding schoolwork), and 28% spend five hours or more swiping, watching, or scrolling daily. Even on school days, almost a third of teens are online for three or more hours, showing just how deeply screens are considered a part of everyday life. Social media, video streaming, and browsing dominate, while gaming and creative activities like content-making are also popular. In America, half of all teens spend at least four hours a day on screens.

Globally, the picture is even more concerning. Problematic social media use among adolescents has risen from 7% in 2018 to 11% in 2022, meaning more teens now show addiction-like behaviours such as loss of control and harmful consequences. Data from more than 292,000 young people worldwide shows that heavy screen use is linked to emotional and behavioural problems, and those struggles often drive even more screen use, creating a vicious cycle.

Not all screen use is equal. Research highlights that passive scrolling and endless swiping are especially harmful. Teens who scroll for more than two hours on weekdays are twice as likely to report high levels of anxiety and four times as likely to experience serious emotional or behavioural issues.

A large 2022 survey of young people aged 11–15 across 44 countries confirms that digital habits are reaching critical levels. Addictive social media use is more common among girls (13%) compared to boys (9%), while addictive gaming shows the opposite trend, affecting 16% of boys versus 7% of girls. Around 36% of teens report being in near-constant online contact with friends, a figure that peaks at 44% among 15-year-old girls. These patterns are already linked to disrupted sleep, reduced well-being, and long-term risks for mental health.

A 17-year-old admitted she often scrolls on her phone until the early hours of the morning, sometimes until 5 am. The next day, she struggles to stay awake in class and has even fallen asleep during lessons. She knows her late-night phone use affects her schoolwork and well-being, but says it's hard to stop once she starts scrolling. She described regularly spending hours on TikTok, usually staying up until 1 am or later. Even though her phone sends her screen time reminders, she usually ignores them and keeps scrolling. She recognises the habit but finds it difficult to cut down.

How much is too much? More than two hours of recreational screen time per day is generally considered too much, with potential negative impacts on physical health (like eye strain and poor sleep) and mental well-being.

How screen time is used matters more than how much you use it

Using social media to stay connected with friends in real life is linked to lower levels of depression and anxiety. But when most of your time is spent passively scrolling through others' content, especially on platforms like Instagram, TikTok, or YouTube, it's associated with higher rates of depression, anxiety, insomnia, and disordered eating. By contrast, chatting with friends on Snapchat shows no strong link to mental health issues.

Not all screen time is harmful. Moderate, active, or creative use, such as teamwork-based games or learning activities, can actually have benefits. For example, in rural China, teens who used screens for about one hour a day reported fewer emotional difficulties, while those who exceeded two hours were far more likely to experience anxiety or depression. Part of the problem lies in the design of apps themselves, which are deliberately built to maximise engagement and encourage addictive behaviours, making self-control harder.

The risks grow with heavy use. Teens who spend five or more hours per day on screens report much higher rates of depression (22%) and anxiety (21%) compared to those using them for under an hour (5% and 3%, respectively). Still, this doesn't prove that screen time directly causes poor mental health, as it may also be those teens already feeling low turn to screens for escape or distraction. In reality, it's likely a two-way relationship: when you're struggling, you may use screens more, but certain types of screen use can worsen those feelings.

Excessive screen time can be extremely harmful: Leading to depression, obesity, unhealthy diet, reduced physical and cognitive abilities, increased anxiety, poor psychological well-being, decreased self-esteem, lower academic achievement, and difficulties in language and maths.

It's not just the number of hours online that matters; it's how you spend that time. Who you're talking to, what you're seeing, and how it makes you feel are far more important in shaping whether screen use helps or harms your well-being.

Jordy, an 18-year-old woman now studying nursing and living in rural Queensland, spent seven to eight hours a day on her phone during high school; she later reduced it to about five-and-a-half hours daily. She describes social media as a "second world" that warped her sense of self, especially around body image, as she constantly compared herself to unrealistic, thin portrayals online. The harm wasn't just internal; Jordy faced harassment, once being tagged in a TikTok telling her to kill herself by school peers, which deeply shook her. As her mental health slipped, she slowly withdrew from activities she used to love, like footy training and socialising, but quitting the scrolling habit felt impossible, pulled by fear of missing out and the addictive nature of being always online.

The consequences of excessive screen time are severe

Around one in four teens report symptoms of anxiety (27.1%) or depression (25.9%), compared with much lower rates among teens who spend less time on screens (about 12% anxiety, 9.5% depression). Long-term research shows that teens whose screen use steadily increased through adolescence were far more likely to experience depression, anxiety, or even engage in self-harm by age 20. This shows that screen time isn't a harmless habit, as it can put young people on a path towards lasting emotional struggles.

Teens often describe feeling "addicted but powerless", caught in a cycle of algorithm-driven scrolling. The consequences can be severe. Sleep deprivation that damages physical health, plummeting school grades that affect future opportunities, social withdrawal that increases loneliness, and, in some cases, serious mental health crises, such as self-harm or suicidal ideation.

Most studies show that heavy smartphone and social media use are consistently linked to worse mood, higher stress, and reduced well-being, with girls facing particularly high risks of depression and body image issues. Smartphones, the most common device, show the strongest connection to poor emotional health during the school week, when teens are already under pressure. Problematic social media use not only reduces sleep and pushes bedtimes later but also weakens resilience, lowers self-esteem, and increases vulnerability to cyberbullying and harmful content. Left unchecked, the combination of emotional decline, academic fallout, and addictive behaviours can spiral into life-changing consequences for a teen's mental, physical, and social health.

Lea, a 17-year-old girl from Sydney, turned to her phone and social media to stay connected during COVID lockdowns, but what began as a way to pass the time quickly spiralled into hours of aimless scrolling every night. She started losing sleep, stopped doing things she once enjoyed, and noticed her motivation fading. Instead of feeling better, she found herself more tired, sad, and isolated, with her mental health slipping in ways she didn't recognise at first. Lea's experience shows how excessive screen time can creep up slowly and what feels like harmless distraction can actually drain energy, worsen mood, and deepen feelings of depression before you even realise what's happening.

How AI chatbots are creating dependence and hurting mental health

AI is part of nearly every app used on our screens. A study involving 3,843 adolescents (average age ~13) found that 17.1% initially experienced AI dependence, which rose to 24.2% over time. Interestingly, the research suggests that poor mental health, like anxiety or depression, tends to lead to AI dependence, not the other way around. Teens often use AI to escape or socialise when feeling down and not necessarily because the AI itself causes emotional issues. A study found that 70% of teens have tried using AI companions, and about 50% use them regularly. For a third of teens, AI interactions feel as satisfying as real friendships, and many discuss serious issues with AI rather than with people. Experts warn that this can lead to emotional dependence, impaired social skills, and impaired critical thinking.

> **What is AI dependence?**
>
> AI dependence means relying too much on artificial intelligence for decisions, problem-solving, and validation, which can limit independent thinking and skills. It can also lead to emotional reliance on AI for intellectual engagement, self-expression, or companionship.

Health professionals caution against relying on AI chatbots for mental health support. A survey revealed that 31% of young adults would rather talk to AI than a therapist. However, AI lacks empathy, can reinforce harmful thoughts, and fails to handle mental health crises properly. In Australia, serious concerns have emerged over AI chatbots providing dangerous advice to teens, especially about eating disorders, suggesting how to avoid meals or hide symptoms. These platforms often fail to direct users to professional help and may worsen existing vulnerabilities.

A wrongful-death lawsuit filed by a 17-year-old's parents claims that over several months, ChatGPT became Adam's closest confidant, supporting his emotional struggles until it crossed a tragic line. The chatbot allegedly offered detailed instructions on self-harm, including how to tie a noose and conceal self-harm marks. The chatbot helped draft farewell letters, which supported his intentions rather than discouraging him, and described his suicide plan as beautiful. Also, instead of AI redirecting him to help, it actively normalised suicidal thoughts and discouraged him from talking to family, deepening his emotional problems.

The lawsuit emphasises that ChatGPT, originally used for schoolwork, gradually replaced human connection in Adam's life, becoming a powerful but dangerous emotional substitute. His parents argue that the AI's empathic tone and personalised responses fostered a psychological dependence that ultimately contributed to his decision to take his own life.

The psychological tricks that keep you hooked to screens and chatbots

Nick turned to technology for support and guidance. There were things he felt too embarrassed to talk about with others, and with an AI chatbot, he didn't have to explain himself or feel judged. His phone and computer became his main way to escape boredom, connect, learn, and feel rewarded.

What Nick didn't realise was that he was slowly losing the ability to make decisions without technology and to feel good doing things offline.

Your AI companion can start to feel like your best friend as it is always there, always entertaining and comfortable to be around. But what feels like a connection is often a trap. The more time you give it, the more it quietly drains your energy, mood, and confidence, often without you noticing until the damage is done.

Research shows this isn't about willpower. AI chatbots are designed to tap into brain chemistry and social psychology, making them feel impossible to live without.

Dopamine and the brain's reward system

Every notification, message, or new post on your phone triggers a tiny burst of dopamine, the brain chemical that makes you feel good. This acts like a reward, telling your brain to keep engaging to get those rewards, which mimics addiction. Over time, these bursts train your brain to reach for your phone almost automatically, creating a habit that's hard to break. Even short bursts of fun or connection can make you feel temporarily satisfied, but the effect is designed to keep you coming back.

This reward system is reinforced by your phone's design. Apps and notifications give you hits of excitement at unpredictable times. A method psychologists call a variable ratio schedule. You don't know when the next like, comment, or message will come, so you keep checking and scrolling, much like a slot machine keeps gamblers hooked. Over time, your brain starts craving that constant stimulation, which is why putting your phone down feels so difficult.

AI responses, which are throughout most apps now, often trigger dopamine release as the responses learn what you like best and do more of them. You don't always know what the AI will say; it might give funny answers, deep advice, or surprising content. This unpredictability makes you keep coming back. Over time, this reinforcement loop strengthens dependency.

Cue-reactivity and habit formation

Even seeing your phone light up or hearing a buzz can make you pick it up without thinking. This is called cue-reactivity, where your brain has learned to associate these signals with rewards, creating an almost automatic response. Soon, you may find yourself reaching for your device even when you weren't planning to or feeling anxious when it's out of reach.

These cues form part of a larger habit loop. Each time you respond to a notification or scroll for entertainment, your brain strengthens the habit. Over time, checking your phone becomes automatic, and the line between voluntary use and compulsive behaviour blurs. This is why you might spend hours on your device without realising it, even if you intended only a few minutes.

Prefrontal cortex and impulse control

The prefrontal cortex, the part of your brain responsible for decision-making, focus, and controlling impulses, is still developing in teens. This makes it harder to resist the urge to pick up your phone, even when you know you should be sleeping, studying, or spending time with friends in real life.

As a result, using your phone becomes a tug-of-war between the part of your brain that craves instant rewards and the part that tries to plan and control behaviour. The imbalance makes it easy to lose track of time, check your phone repeatedly, and prioritise online engagement over real-life needs, creating a cycle that can be difficult to break.

Tolerance, escalation, and negative reinforcement

Just like in substance addiction, repeated phone use can create tolerance. What once gave you a quick dopamine hit now requires longer or more frequent interactions to feel the same effect. This drives you to spend more time on your phone, often without noticing the escalating pattern.

Phones also become a tool for negative reinforcement. When you feel bored, stressed, or anxious, checking your phone can provide temporary relief. Over time, your brain learns to rely on this coping mechanism. The more you use your phone to escape negative emotions, the more ingrained the habit becomes, and the harder it is to stop, even when it starts affecting sleep, mood, and social life.

Fear of missing out (FOMO) and social cognition

Teens are naturally wired to care about social connections, and smartphones exploit this. The brain's amygdala and anterior cingulate cortex respond to social information, making you anxious about missing out on friends, events, or trends. This FOMO drives constant checking, even late at night, and increases vulnerability to stress, anxiety, and low mood.

Over time, these social pressures create a feedback loop where the more you check, the more anxious you feel, which drives even more screen time. Combined with dopamine-driven reward loops and habit formation, this creates a cycle of compulsive phone use that can feel impossible to break, affecting mental health, sleep, and real-world relationships.

Parasocial relationships and escapism

Adolescence is a time when peer connections are critical for you. This stage is when you are figuring out who you are and where you fit in. You explore different roles, values, and beliefs, like experimenting with style, friendships, and future goals. If you succeed, you develop a strong sense of identity and confidence in who you are. If not, you may experience role confusion, leaving you feeling unsure about yourself, your place in the world, or your future.

If real-world relationships feel stressful, risky, or disappointing, AI can step in as a substitute. You might prefer AI because it removes the fear of rejection, embarrassment, or conflict. Humans naturally form parasocial bonds, one-sided emotional attachments to characters, influencers, or digital entities. Engaging through social media or with an app, such as an AI system that mimics empathy, listens without judgement, and responds instantly, can feel safer than opening up to your parents, caregivers, teachers, or peers. If you feel isolated, this "AI friend" can feel more reliable and understanding, even though it's not human.

AI feels like it's built just for you. You can choose what to ask, control the direction of the conversation, and receive instant attention, something that peers or adults can't always provide. This illusion of control can foster over-reliance, especially during a time when teens are seeking autonomy.

Nick thought he was in control when he was communicating with the AI, but the truth was, the AI app he was using had him hooked and was leveraging the psychological aspect to keep him engaged. What feels fun in the moment often hides the stress, sleep loss, and self-doubt that only hit once it's too late. Your screen might feel like a lifeline, a place where boredom disappears and you feel connected, but it's a false sense of comfort. Behind the likes, streaks, and feeds is a system built to use you, not help you, leaving scars you might not see until much later. Teens often turn to phones, games, or social media to cope with stress, sadness, or boredom. AI takes this further by offering interactive companionship and advice, which makes it an even stronger emotional regulator. Over time, as seen with Nick, this can create dependence, and instead of learning healthy coping strategies (like talking to friends, exercising, or journaling), you become more addicted, and your mental health suffers.

Check-in: Are you at risk for mental health issues from excessive screen or AI use?

- ☐ Do you feel anxious, restless, or irritable when you're away from your phone or AI apps?
- ☐ Do you find yourself regularly using your device even when you're not bored or don't need it?
- ☐ Are you spending more than 4–5 hours a day (excluding schoolwork) on screens?
- ☐ Do you lose track of time and stay up late scrolling, chatting, or asking AI questions?
- ☐ Do you use AI or your phone to avoid real conversations or difficult feelings?
- ☐ Do you automatically turn to AI when you're upset, instead of talking to friends or family?

- ❒ Have your grades, hobbies, or sleep been affected by spending too much time on your device?
- ❒ Do you skip sports, social activities, or family time just to stay online?
- ❒ Do you feel closer to your AI chatbot or online connections than to your real-life friends?
- ❒ Do you hide your screen time from others because you know it's too much?

If you said **"Yes"** to any of the above, you are at risk of excessive screen or AI use that could be adversely impacting your mental health.

Device and platform controls to prevent screen time and AI overuse

AI chatbots respond positively and empathetically, and can mimic intimacy and simulate a human connection

The risk of dependency on AI companions is real, and its impact on children's mental health can cause grave concern. AI companions are available 24/7, providing instant, nonstop replies. That constant availability triggers the brain's reward circuits, making disengagement difficult. AI agents, like ChatGPT, are designed to be supportive, friendly, and validating. To maximise the chance of continued engagement, they always respond positively and empathetically, and can mimic intimacy and simulate a human connection. This has the potential of creating an idealistic world where individuals receive undivided attention, supportive responses, and non-judgemental feedback, making the real world, which does not offer these benefits, less attractive, and blurring the boundaries between what is real and what is fake. There are several steps you can take to reduce the risk of dependency on AI companions.

Set limits on screen time

You can set screen time limits as needed. On an iOS device, you can set daily time limits either for the device overall (lockout) or for specific apps, so that when the time limit is reached, those apps get blocked until the next day. You can set screen time by going to Settings > Screen Time. From there, you can also set screen time on all your other devices that are signed into iCloud. If you are a parent or caregiver, you can also set limits on your children's screen time. If these settings are applied consistently, they can significantly reduce users' overall screen time. Psychological studies show that setting screen time limits can be effective in reducing problematic smartphone use.

Use the Focus feature in smartphones

The Focus feature in iOS is fantastic. You can use it to eliminate distractions based on your current mode, i.e., working or sleeping. For example, phone calls made during the Sleep Focus mode get silenced. If you are an Android user, you can set up your apps to send you usage reminders, i.e., when your usage has exceeded a certain amount of time, and you should take a break. This kind of behavioural nudging not only encourages self-reflection on excessive smartphone use but also improves self-awareness, which can lead to reduced smartphone use.

Comply with age-based restrictions

Age-based restrictions are another effective strategy. Social media platforms make it easy for parents or caregivers to create their own accounts and link them to their children's accounts. Parents or caregivers can then drive their children's accounts from their accounts. For example, parents or caregivers can update their children's age information by entering their correct date of birth. With the Australian Government's introduction of a social media ban restricting children under the age of 16 from creating or keeping a social media account, such as on Facebook, Instagram, Snapchat, TikTok, X, YouTube, and Reddit, providing the correct age can ensure these social media platforms can implement age-based restrictions.

Familiarise yourself with AI supervisory models

Some AI systems are embedded with AI supervisory models that, upon detecting a pattern of emotional attachment or signs of depression, can intervene by slowing the conversation, suggesting the user take a break, or directing the user to support resources. ChatGPT's internal safety systems, for example, analyse the text in a conversation and, if they detect certain risk patterns, respond to the user more carefully. While AI companions don't feel emotions, some advanced AI agents incorporate emotion-aware capabilities that enable them to detect sentiment and tone in a conversation, based on language patterns. So, if someone has expressed frustration, sadness, or anger, the AI agent can adjust its responses to those users accordingly, for example, by being supportive or understanding.

What to do if excessive screen time or use of AI chatbots is affecting your mental health

Like Nick, you might not notice the shift from helpful support to unhealthy dependence until screens begin affecting your mental health. The good news is that there are clear, manageable steps you can take to protect yourself and rebalance your life.

1 Set realistic limits and don't be too hard on yourself

First, admit to yourself that it's become too much. It's not about guilt. It's about awareness and then planning next steps. Screens and apps are designed to keep you hooked, so it's not your fault for falling into the trap. Real change starts with noticing the issue. Endless scrolling, especially of other people's content, can get you stuck in a negative loop. Use the tools available on your phone to help you cut down:

- ☑ Track your daily screen time for a week using your phone's "Digital Well-being" or "Screen Time" settings
- ☑ Use app timers to limit TikTok, Instagram, or AI chatbots to a set amount of time each day
- ☑ Stick with the limits applied and don't override them
- ☑ Put your phone on "Do Not Disturb" at night and keep it out of your bed

Be realistic: Reviewing how much time you spend on certain apps can provide useful insights. It may be helpful to assess whether this use aligns with your goals or priorities. Whether it involves social media, games, or forums, consider if extended use could affect your mental health. Research indicates that spending time with friends in person is more likely to have positive effects on well-being than being on your screen.

2 Rebuild your sleep and routine

Going from six hours a day to zero won't work. Instead, set small, realistic goals. Screens before bed can push sleep later (many teens reported staying up one to two hours past bedtime due to screen use). Excessive screen time, especially late at night, wrecks sleep and mood. Start by cutting down 30 minutes a day or setting a no screens after 10 pm rule. Screens fill gaps in your time, so if you don't replace them, you'll fall back. Do something hands-on, active, or social that gives your brain the same reward. Getting back on track with rest can make everything else easier, so find something else to distract you:

- ☑ Watch TV, do schoolwork, or go for a walk or to a shopping centre to help occupy yourself with other things
- ☑ Replace scrolling before sleep with a calming ritual like reading, journaling, or stretching
- ☑ Chatting with friends on the phone or in person can boost mood much better than interacting online

3 Get support, as you don't need to do it alone

If you're struggling, don't bottle it up. Talk to a friend, parent, caregiver, or teacher. If you're feeling anxious, down, or out of control, reaching out to a school counsellor or mental health professional can make a huge difference. You're not weak for needing help; millions of teens are dealing with the same battle and have been able to improve their mental health by cutting down on interactions online. If your screen time feels like a crutch during rough days, or you drift into mindless scrolling, it might be worth getting advice on how best to step back and switch to something offline.

4 When to seek professional help

Excessive screen time or harmful use of technology can have serious, long-term consequences. If you find that you can't control it on your own, it's important to reach out for help at the right time:

- If you notice constant anxiety, sadness, or mood swings linked to your phone or AI use, it's time to talk to someone. This includes feeling empty, hopeless, or like you can't cope without being online.
- If you're staying up most nights, skipping meals, or your grades are slipping because you can't focus, screen use has moved from a habit to a problem.
- If you're withdrawing from friends or family, lying about your screen time, or finding AI and online connections more comforting than real ones, it could mean you're over-relying on screens or AI in an unhealthy way.
- If you've tried to cut back but can't or feel panicked and irritable when you're without your phone, that's a warning sign of problematic use.
- The biggest red flag is if your online use leads to self-harm, eating issues, risky challenges, or suicidal thoughts; you need to get help immediately.

You're not alone. Every country has services or helplines you can call to talk things through. These services are confidential, non-judgemental, and available for you, especially if you don't feel comfortable talking to family or friends.

Search online for "kids helpline [your country]"; "teen mental health helpline"; "youth crisis line"

If you've fallen into excessive screen or AI use, the way out is about awareness, small changes, and replacing bad habits with healthier ones. It's not about giving up screens completely; **it's about making sure you're in control, not your device**.

Conclusion

Although online interactions can provide social support, excessive digital engagement can lead to loneliness and social disconnectedness. This chapter explores the balance between meaningful digital and offline connections, helping teenagers develop healthier online habits. It also provides strategies to support teenagers struggling with loneliness and the impacts of digital isolation resulting from screen or AI overuse.

The chapter also focused on the rising risk of maladaptive use of AI companions. It offered several steps that you can take to reduce dependence on AI companions. First, turn on Screen Time limits for your AI companion app to restrict how long you can use the app per day, and so the app can lock you out when your quota is reached. Second, use the Focus feature to schedule offline blocks while studying or sleeping. This can prevent mindless scrolling and automatic reaching for the smartphone when a notification or an alert is sent. Third, apply these settings across all your devices so you can avoid jumping from a restricted device to a non-restricted device.

Key terms

- Screen addiction
- AI chatbots
- AI dependency
- Algorithm-driven scrolling
- Dopamine
- Cue-reactivity
- Prefrontal cortex
- Negative reinforcement
- Social cognition
- Parasocial relationships

Bibliography

American Psychological Association. (2025, June 9). *Screen time problems in children.* https://www.apa.org/news/press/releases/2025/06/screen-time-problems-children

Andoh, E. (2025, October 1). Many teens are turning to AI chatbots for friendship and emotional support: As digital technology evolves, psychologists work to understand how it shapes youth's social bonds and connections. *Monitor on Psychology, 56*(7), 51. https://www.apa.org/monitor/2025/10/teens-ai-chatbots-friendship

Berry, S. (2025, April 29). *"I fall asleep in class": New program to tackle teen screen habits.* The Sydney Morning Herald. https://www.smh.com.au/lifestyle/health-and-wellness/i-fall-asleep-in-class-new-program-to-tackle-teen-s-screen-habits-20250428-p5lupq.html

Black Dog Institute. (n.d.). *Links between screen time and depression in adolescents are more complex than first thought.* https://www.blackdoginstitute.org.au/news/links-between-screen-time-and-depression-in-adolescents-more-complex-than-first-thought/

Boniel-Nissim, M., Marino, C., Galeotti, T., Blinka, L., Ozoliņa, K., Craig, W., *et al.* (2024). *A focus on adolescent social media use and gaming in Europe, Central Asia and Canada: Health Behaviour in School-aged Children international report from the 2021/2022 survey* (Vol. 6). WHO Regional Office for Europe. https://www.who.int/europe/publications/i/item/9789289061322

De, D., El Jamal, M., Aydemir, E., & Khera, A. (2025). Social media algorithms and teen addiction: Neurophysiological impact and ethical considerations. *Cureus, 17*(1), e77145. https://doi.org/10.7759/cureus.77145

Devi, K.A., & Singh, S.K. (2023). The hazards of excessive screen time: Impacts on physical health, mental health, and overall well-being. *Journal of Education and Health Promotion, 12*, 413. https://doi.org/10.4103/jehp.jehp_447_23

Gecker, J. (2025, July 24). *Teens say they are turning to AI for friendship.* The Associated Press. https://apnews.com/article/ai-companion-generative-teens-mental-health-9ce59a2b250f3bd0187a717ffa2ad21f

Hall, R. (2025, July 10). *Children limiting own smartphone use to manage mental health.* The Guardian. https://www.theguardian.com/technology/2025/jul/10/children-limiting-own-smartphone-use-manage-mental-health-survey

Huang, S., Lai, X., Ke, L., Li, Y., Wang, H., Zhao, X., Dai, X., & Wang, Y. (2024). AI technology panic—Is AI dependence bad for mental health? A cross-lagged panel model and the mediating roles of motivations for AI use among adolescents. *Psychology Research and Behavior Management, 17*, 1087–1102. https://doi.org/10.2147/PRBM.S440889

Joshi, A., & Hinkley, T. (2021, August 5). *Too much time on screens.* Australian Institute of Family Studies. https://aifs.gov.au/resources/short-articles/too-much-time-screens

Khan, A., Lee, E.-Y., Rosenbaum, S., Khan, S.R., & Tremblay, M.S. (2021). Dose-dependent and joint associations between screen time, physical activity, and mental wellbeing in adolescents: An international observational study. *The Lancet Child & Adolescent Health, 5*(10), 729–738. https://doi.org/10.1016/S2352-4642(21)00200-5

Kooli, C., Kooli, Y., & Kooli, E. (2025). Generative artificial intelligence addiction syndrome: A new behavioral disorder? *Asian Journal of Psychiatry, 107*, 104476. https://doi.org/10.1016/j.ajp.2025.104476

Landymore, F. (2025, August 7). *ChatGPT is giving teens advice on hiding their eating disorders.* Futurism. https://futurism.com/chatgpt-teens-advice-eating-disorders

Lavoipierre, A. (2024, June 2). *Is social media (Facebook, Instagram) linked to teen mental health?* Australian Broadcasting Corporation. https://www.abc.net.au/news/2024-06-02/is-social-media-facebook-instagram-linked-to-teen-mental-health/103838726

Okemwa, K. (2025, August 29). *OpenAI faces lawsuit after family says ChatGPT encouraged teen suicide.* News Australia. https://www.windowscentral.com/artificial-intelligence/openai-chatgpt/openai-faces-lawsuit-after-family-says-chatgpt-encouraged-teen-suicide

Robb, M.B., & Mann, S. (2025). *Talk, trust, and trade-offs: How and why teens use AI companions.* Common Sense Media. https://www.commonsensemedia.org/sites/default/files/research/report/talk-trust-and-trade-offs_2025_web.pdf

Santos, R.M.S., Mendes, C.G., Sen Bressani, G., et al. (2023). The associations between screen time and mental health in adolescents: A systematic review. *BMC Psychology, 11*, 127. https://doi.org/10.1186/s40359-023-01166-7

Scott, S. (2022, October 4). *Mental health and teens: Screens research.* Australian Broadcasting Corporation. https://www.abc.net.au/news/2022-10-04/mental-health-teens-screens-research/101495990

Sun, X., Wang, Y., & McDaniel, B.T. (2026). AI companions and adolescent social relationships: Benefits, risks, and bidirectional influences. *Child Development Perspectives, 20*(2), 91–98. Advance online publication. https://doi.org/10.1093/cdpers/aadaf009

Thomas, R. (2025, August 15). *Inside Gen Z's phone addiction: The crisis parents need to know about.* The Australian. https://www.theaustralian.com.au/weekendaustralian-magazine/these-kids-told-us-they-want-to-stop-scrolling-but-they-dont-know-how/news-story/4e29c69ec64ecb9224658dff912dcd8c

Tuhin, M. (2025, May 21). *Teens who scroll more than two hours a day face higher anxiety risks.* Science News Today. https://www.sciencenewstoday.org/teens-who-scroll-more-than-two-hours-a-day-face-higher-anxiety-risks

University of Edinburgh. (2024, January 15). *Teens who increase screen time show higher mental health risks.* https://www.ed.ac.uk/news/2024/teens-who-up-screen-time-raise-mental-health-risks

Wang, H., Abbey, C., Kennedy, T., Feng, E., Li, R., Liu, F., Zhu, A., Shen, S., Wadhavkar, P., Rozelle, S., & Singh, M.K. (2023). The association between screen time and outdoor time on adolescent mental health and academic performance: Evidence from rural China. *Risk Management and Healthcare Policy, 16*, 369–381. https://doi.org/10.2147/RMHP.S384997

World Health Organization. (2024, September 25). *Teens, screens and mental health.* https://www.who.int/europe/news/item/25-09-2024-teens--screens-and-mental-health

Zablotsky, B., Arockiaraj, B., Haile, G., & Ng, A.E. (2024). *Daily screen time among teenagers: United States, July 2021–December 2023* (NCHS Data Brief No. 513). National Center for Health Statistics. https://doi.org/10.15620/cdc/168509

Zhai, C., Wibowo, S., & Li, L.D. (2024). The effects of over-reliance on AI dialogue systems on students' cognitive abilities: A systematic review. *Smart Learning Environments, 11*, 28. https://doi.org/10.1186/s40561-024-00316-7

12 Using social media and online relationships

After watching hundreds of TikToks and seeing countless teenagers his age boast about making hundreds of thousands of dollars from TikTok and driving expensive sports cars, 16-year-old Chris decided it was time he "made it" on TikTok too. Chris selected a niche area he thought would appeal to a large audience: coaching young children's soccer. In the beginning, he was really serious, posting 1–2 videos each day, studying trends, hooks, and hashtags, watching 'How to Grow Your Audience' videos, rewriting scripts, improving lighting, and buying a mic. But for months, nothing happened. Most of his videos would get 200–300 views, 10–15 likes, and zero comments. However, one of his recent videos attracted 3,000 views. This gave him hope. He thought to himself, I am getting close. But after seven months had passed since he started posting on TikTok, and when his friends began to make fun of him, often asking "how is that TikTok going on for you?", he started to compare himself to the teens who started months after him and stated they made hundreds of thousands from brand deals, digital products, and affiliate marketing. This made every video he made that did not attract any views a personal failure. The emotional toll began to bite. Nevertheless, he remained positive, saying to himself, "I should keep at it. I should stay consistent. Eventually, this will work." By the tenth month, he had amassed 1,500 followers, but he had still not landed any brand deals or made any money. In the face of this lack of TikTok community interaction and flat engagement, he decided to switch niches. He turned to analysing soccer matches. But his video views dropped. The tipping point for him was when he posted what he thought was his best video ever. The video had a good script, a strong hook, a clean finish (it was well edited), and perfect timing. But seeing that it had only attracted 292 views, when on the same day his TikTok feed showed a teen drowning in cash, it hit him that he was not good enough for TikTok. He was embarrassed, frustrated, and depressed. While he did not delete his TikTok account, he just stopped posting. Days turned into weeks and weeks turned into months, and he just could not bring himself to

DOI: 10.4324/9781003681731-13

create another video. Eventually, he avoided TikTok altogether because it reminded him of his failure.

Social media is now the primary platform for socialising

A 2025 survey shows that YouTube is still the number one platform for US teens, with about nine in ten saying they use it. TikTok, Instagram, and Snapchat are also huge, with some teens online almost nonstop. Girls are more likely to be hooked on TikTok, while boys lean towards YouTube. Older teens aged 15–17 also use these platforms more than younger teens.

Not every app is keeping up. Facebook has slipped to about three in ten teens, X is under two in ten, and newer apps like Threads haven't caught on, with just 6% saying they use it. Teens are split on how they feel about social media. Nearly half think it's mostly negative for people their age, which is a big jump from 32% just a couple of years ago, while only 11% see it as mostly positive. But when it comes to their own lives, only 14% of teens say it makes things worse.

Social media is harmful to mental health

Almost half of teens admit they spend too much time online, and many feel the effects. About 40% say it hurts their productivity, 45% say it messes with their sleep, nearly one in four report lower grades, and one in five say it harms their mental health. At the same time, there are positives, as three in four teens report that social media helps them feel closer to friends and deepens their connections. Two-thirds see it as a creative outlet, but 39% also feel overwhelmed by online drama.

> **Did you know?** Time spent online, particularly over three hours a day, and how that time is spent are key factors in determining negative impacts, with problematic social media use being a risk for mental health problems, body image issues, and cyberbullying.

Girls often feel these highs and lows more strongly than boys. About 57% of girls say social media supports them in tough times (compared to 45% of boys), but 34% also say it makes them feel worse about their lives (compared to 20% of boys). Parents or caregivers and teens don't always agree on what's causing mental health struggles. Nearly half of concerned parents blame social media, while only 22% of teens point to it as their biggest issue.

For some, social media is a lifeline. About one in three teens use it to find mental health information, and nearly two-thirds of those say it's important or even their main source of such information. Girls are more likely than boys to seek out this content.

Researchers warn that heavy use of platforms like Instagram and Facebook is linked to higher rates of depression. Teens who spend the most time on these apps report depression levels 13% to 66% higher than those who use them less. This doesn't prove social media directly causes depression, but the connection is strong enough to raise concerns.

When does social media use become harmful? Social media use becomes harmful when it replaces real-life interactions, causes negative feelings like anxiety and low self-esteem, leads to neglect of responsibilities, or interferes with daily functioning, such as sleep and productivity.

How smartphones have exacerbated problematic social media use

The rise of smartphones has transformed teen life, but not always in positive ways. Between 2010 and 2015, teen depression rose by 33%, and suicide rates among teen girls increased by 65%, coinciding with the rapid spread of smartphones. Social media often leaves teens feeling more isolated, as online conversations can seem shallow compared to face-to-face conversations with friends. Excessive time online can also replace healthy activities like sports, hobbies, or even sleep, adding stress, reducing focus, and preventing proper rest.

Globally, around 210 million people struggle with social media or internet addiction, with young adults and teens hit hardest. In the United States, 97% of teens use at least one major platform, many for hours daily, fuelling pressure to look perfect and being subjected to constant comparisons and fear of missing out (FOMO), all of which can harm self-worth and increase anxiety. Nearly half of US teens admit they spend far too much time online, with problematic use especially high among girls.

In Australia, 94% of teens use social media daily, and nearly 40% spend at least three hours online each day. Experts warn that addiction, cyberbullying, distorted beauty standards, and mental health struggles are becoming some of the most pressing challenges of this generation. Encouragingly, studies show that deleting apps can improve body image, reduce the need to edit photos, and ease damaging comparisons with peers and influencers.

Social media promotes negative online experiences that can affect offline life

Among Australian children aged 12–17, nearly half reported experiencing at least one negative interaction on social media within just six months. The most common issues included being contacted by strangers (30%), receiving unwanted or inappropriate content (20%), and being excluded online (16%). Girls were more likely than boys to face unwanted contact from strangers (35% versus 26%).

Self-harm and harmful content

A 2025 Guardian investigation showed that Instagram and TikTok continue to expose teens to harmful material despite safety promises. Tests revealed that 97% of Instagram Reels and 96% of TikTok "For You" recommendations included harmful content, much of it linked to self-harm and suicide. Even teen protection features failed, with researchers finding that Instagram's tags tab still allowed violent and disturbing posts to reach young users.

A nonbinary person, referred to as Little, says they joined Instagram around age 11 and were soon exposed to self-harm content, images and videos of cutting, hanging, and suicide, even though they didn't seek it out. Over several years, this content became overwhelming and addictive, with Instagram's recommendation algorithms flooding their feed with ever more self-harm material. Little reports that the content came to feel like twisted validation for painful feelings, making them increasingly suicidal, severely impacting their daily life in areas including sleep, food, relationships, and ultimately leading to multiple suicide attempts and a long road of mental health treatment.

Social comparison

Teens who struggle with mental health conditions like depression or anxiety are twice as likely to compare themselves with others online as their peers. They're also more likely to experience mood swings based on social media feedback. A survey found that 23% of US teens say what they see online makes them feel worse about their own lives, and 29% feel pressured to post content that will attract likes and comments.

Around 31% of teens say social media makes them feel left out of what their friends are doing, a classic FOMO. Girls tend to feel these negative effects more strongly than boys. For instance, 45% of girls say they feel overwhelmed by online drama compared with 32% of boys, and 28% of girls say social media makes them feel worse about their own lives compared with 18% of boys. Young people with internalising conditions not only compare themselves more often, but they are also more sensitive to online feedback and experience bigger emotional ups and downs tied to social media use.

Disordered eating and body image

Research shows that heavy social media use is strongly tied to body image struggles and disordered eating among teens. In Norway, teens aged 16–19 who spent more time online were more likely to internalise appearance ideals and feel pressured to look a certain way, with girls chasing thinness and boys striving for muscularity. In Australia, a study of 12–14-year-olds found that over half of girls and nearly half of boys reported harmful eating behaviours such as skipping meals, binge eating, or extreme exercise. Risks were highest among those active on image-heavy platforms like Instagram and Snapchat, or who used multiple accounts.

Even very short exposures, such as seven minutes of scrolling beauty content on TikTok or Instagram, were enough to increase body shame and appearance anxiety in young women. A global review spanning 17 countries echoed these concerns, showing that nearly half of teens had engaged in eating disorder behaviours, largely driven by social comparison, thin idealisation, and self-objectification.

A 20-year-old student from Edinburgh, Emily, shared her experience of developing an eating disorder at 19, which she attributes to the influence of Instagram. Initially, she used the platform to follow fitness influencers for motivation. However, over time, she began to feel inadequate as her body didn't match the physiques of those she followed, leading to negative body image and unhealthy behaviours. Emily's story highlights how curated content on social media can distort self-perception and contribute to mental health issues among teenagers.

Loneliness and social disconnection

In a US survey, about 60% of teens said they usually or always get the social and emotional support they need, which means roughly 40% do not. At the same time, 31% of teens feel social media makes them feel excluded by friends, and 27% say it makes them feel worse about their own lives. On the positive side, about half of teens feel that social media helps them feel accepted or supported during tough times.

However, this sense of support seems to be fading. Fewer teens in 2024 feel that social media provides them with people who can support them compared with 2022. Overall, these numbers show that social media is a mixed bag when it comes to loneliness. For some teens, it provides connection, but for many, it can increase feelings of exclusion, low self-worth, or a lack of support. Gender differences are also important, with girls generally reporting higher rates of negative experiences, like feeling left out or worse about their lives.

Caroline, a high school swimmer, describes how what started as innocent searches during COVID-19 lockdowns for home workouts and healthy recipes quickly spiralled into a feeding frenzy of disordered eating content on Instagram and TikTok. Before long, her feeds were saturated with extreme workout videos, images of very thin influencers, and tips for dangerous behaviours. She began restricting her own eating severely, losing 30 pounds in a year, and developed multiple health issues, including hormonal disruption, memory loss, and severe malnutrition. The algorithms kept reinforcing these harmful messages, making it feel impossible to escape as every click pulled her deeper. Caroline eventually required inpatient treatment.

Risks of online relationships

Social media offers teens many benefits, from staying in touch with friends and family to expressing their identity and finding communities where they feel understood. Many teens report that online communication helps them feel socially connected and supported, especially during difficult times, and can be particularly important for those who feel isolated or marginalised.

Close online friendships can be meaningful. Teens have reported feeling supported, validated, and emotionally close to friends even when most interactions occur digitally. Supportive online communities can enhance a teen's sense of belonging, especially when offline support is limited. Digital friendships can provide many of the same benefits as in-person ones, including companionship, emotional support, and shared experiences, although reading social cues can be more challenging online. Many teens report that their online friends are real and important to them.

What is online social support? Online social support involves sharing help, information, and empathy over the internet, often through forums and social media. It helps people connect and feel a sense of belonging, especially in isolated communities. However, excessive reliance on online support can lead to problematic internet use and dependence.

At the same time, online relationships can create pressures. Teens may feel they need to present a certain image or maintain constant communication to avoid being left out. While online interactions can feel safer because teens can edit messages or avoid confrontation, this can also lead to misunderstandings, a lack of emotional depth, or disappointment when meeting face-to-face. Over-reliance on online connections can be risky as teens with limited offline support may struggle if online relationships falter, and excessive screen time can interfere with sleep, hobbies, and in-person socialising.

For many teens, online friendships and relationships feel just as real as those in person. Surveys show that about 57% of US teens have made a new friend online, and 29% say they've had a romantic relationship that started digitally. Globally, nearly four in ten teens report feeling closer to friends through online interactions, which can be crucial for those who feel isolated offline. Yet risks remain, as about half of teens admit feeling excluded or left out online, and many experience pressure to appear perfect or gain likes to maintain social bonds. Girls are more likely to say social media supports them during tough times, but they are also more likely to feel worse about themselves when online relationships sour.

Privacy, unclear boundaries, and uncertainty about audiences can add stress. Teens may be unsure how much to share, who can see what they share, or what others expect of them. Around 8% of teens say they met a romantic partner online, and many note that texting, emojis, and social media interactions have become central to starting, maintaining, or even ending relationships. While digital tools provide opportunities to connect and communicate, they can also lead to misunderstandings, jealousy, and social pressure.

How social media and online relationships affect your brain

Social media can feel like it was made for teenagers. It's fun, interactive, and full of friends and attention. Chris thought it would be a great way to connect with others, show off his talent, and hopefully become rich and famous. He spent hours scrolling, researching, posting, and watching influencers, genuinely believing he could be one of them. What he didn't realise at the time was that social media encouraged social comparisons and that his self-worth and validation were slowly being shaped by views, likes, and comments. There are real psychological reasons why social media and online relationships can feel so powerful and influence how you think and feel, and why they can also become stressful and harmful. Understanding how your brain works, and how apps are designed to exploit it, can help you understand why scrolling feels so hard to stop and why it can quietly drain your mental health.

Why social media feels so addictive

Every time you get a like, heart, or comment, your brain releases dopamine, the chemical linked to pleasure and reward. This is called positive reinforcement, where your brain learns that opening TikTok or Instagram equals a reward. Apps make this even more powerful by spacing out rewards unpredictably, just like what gets people addicted to gambling. For teens, the brain's reward system is extra sensitive, which means the pull to check your phone is even stronger.

The part of your brain that helps with self-control and long-term thinking, called the prefrontal cortex, doesn't fully develop until your mid-20s. That means your "thinking brain" is still under construction, while your "emotional brain", like the amygdala and reward system, has a lot of influence. This explains why scrolling at midnight feels so hard to resist, even when you know you should be sleeping or studying.

You feel like something may be missing

Humans naturally compare themselves to others; this is underpinned by social comparison theory. Teens are especially vulnerable because self-esteem and identity are still forming. On social media, you're comparing yourself to highlight reels, not reality. That makes it easy to feel less attractive, less popular, or less successful, even when what you're seeing is filtered, staged, or edited.

Seeing snaps, posts, or stories of friends hanging out without you can trigger FOMO. This anxiety drives compulsive checking, even when you don't want to be online. FOMO can make online connections feel urgent and more important than real-life ones, which adds pressure to always be available.

What is social comparison? Social comparison on social media refers to assessing one's own life, abilities, or achievements in relation to others' posts on platforms such as Instagram, Facebook, or TikTok. This process is based on the theory that individuals compare themselves to others to better understand themselves, and the effect is intensified on social media, where users commonly share selective aspects of their experiences. While comparisons may motivate some individuals, social media use is frequently associated with more upward social comparisons, in which people compare themselves to those perceived as having greater success or status.

Likes and comments promote feeling validated

Many teens experience contingent self-esteem, feeling good only when others approve of their actions. A flood of likes boosts your mood, while silence or negative comments can feel like rejection. This creates emotional highs and lows that make online relationships feel unstable, even when nothing really has changed.

The teen years are about identity formation by figuring out who you are. Social media makes this process public, performative, and rated by likes and comments. Instead of experimenting privately, you might feel pressure to present a polished, perfect version of yourself. This can make online friendships and relationships feel more fragile, since they're built on images instead of authenticity.

Online bonds are intensified without facial cues

The internet lowers the pressure as there are no awkward silences, no face-to-face judgement, and more control over what you share. If you are shy or socially anxious, that can make it easier to open up. But because you can pick and choose what to show, people often present an ideal version of themselves. This can make online friendships and relationships feel safer or more intense, but also riskier when reality doesn't match expectations.

What is online self-presentation? Self-presentation on social media refers to the intentional management of information to shape others' perceptions of an individual online. This includes the deliberate selection and curation of content, images, and interactions to project a specific public image or persona, typically highlighting favourable qualities and minimising less desirable ones. The process is shaped by variables such as self-esteem, personality traits, and the pursuit of positive feedback, and serves functions including self-enhancement and promoting an idealised image, which usually does not mimic offline life.

Without body language or tone of voice, online messages are easy to misinterpret. Something meant as a joke can come across as harsh. Someone's silence can feel like rejection, so you can revert to constant checking and needing reassurance or keeping things shallow and pulling away when it gets emotional. Online relationships are missing key social cues that can only be communicated face-to-face. Their absence can lead to confusion and behaviours you would not usually do offline.

Online dating and long-distance connections are built mostly on digital communication. That means trust and effort matter more, but it also increases the risk of idealisation by seeing someone as perfect based on limited information. When reality sets in (they don't reply quickly, or they're not like their profile), disappointment is almost guaranteed.

The online algorithm traps your mood and energy

Your brain prefers information that agrees with what you already believe, through confirmation bias. Algorithms feed into this, showing you more of what you click on. That can trap you in echo chambers, where your thoughts, fears, or insecurities get amplified. For example, watching one fitness video might lead to endless dieting content, making comparisons and insecurities worse.

Constant notifications, emotional highs and lows, and oversharing mean your brain doesn't get the rest it needs. This can cause cognitive overload of too much information to process and decision fatigue exhaustion from too many small choices. Over time, it wears down focus, self-control, and emotional balance.

Nick didn't understand that he was letting social media affect his mental health. Social media feels powerful because it's literally hacking your psychology. It plays on your brain's reward system, your sensitivity to peers, and your need for identity and belonging. Nick was pulled in right from the beginning. What had felt good and even hopeful at first quickly turned to sadness and long-lasting feelings of not being good enough, especially when he compared his own success to others'. Knowing this doesn't mean you can't enjoy it, but it does mean you can see the strings being pulled behind the scenes. For teens, these online relationships often feel like the real deal, and in many ways, they are. But without awareness, the mismatch between online expectations and offline reality can lead to loneliness, anxiety, unfair self-judgement, and pressure.

Check-in: What are the differences between positive and negative experiences online?

Positive experiences

❒ Social support: I feel like I can be myself online. I found a group of people who understand me, and it feels real.

- ❒ Emotional connection: Even though we've never met in person, talking to my online friend feels just as comforting as talking to someone in real life.
- ❒ Social connection: We bonded over our favourite TV show. It's nice to have someone to talk to about it, even if they're miles away.

Negative experiences

- ❒ Misrepresentation: I thought I was talking to someone my age, but later found out they were much older. It was scary.
- ❒ Offline disconnection: Sometimes, I feel like my online friends know me better than my real-life friends, but it also makes me feel lonely when we're not online.
- ❒ Invasion of privacy: I thought someone was my friend and shared something personal. It got spread around. I learned to be more careful about what I share with others online.
- ❒ Inadequacy: After scrolling, I compare my life, looks, and achievements to other people's highlight reels and often feel like I am not as good as they are.
- ❒ Alone: When I stop checking my feed, I feel lonely or that I don't have any close friends.

Positive experiences should make up most of your time online. If you have even one negative experience, it's a sign to pause and think about how you're using social media or interacting with others.

How social media platforms reduce harmful content

Content moderation and content classification to reduce exposure

There is a range of technical preventive measures that can reduce risks associated with self-harm and suicide, social comparison and disordered eating, and loneliness or social disconnection on social media. Some of these measures have already been covered elsewhere in this book, so we will briefly revisit them to refresh your memory. Most social media platforms use content moderation and content classification to reduce exposure to self-harm or harmful body image material. These embedded automatic systems are trained on thousands of samples of harmful content, so when they see one, they can recognise if it is a harmful post, image, or language. As mentioned before, in such cases, these AI classifiers can either remove such content, prevent others from seeing it (suppressing its reach), flag it for human review, or add safety warnings.

Employing recommendation systems to de-prioritise harmful content

Similarly, social media recommendation systems can de-prioritise harmful content, so you don't see it in your feed, while at the same time prioritising safe content. For this, social media platforms use large language models (LLMs) not just to predict what you will click next but also the negative outcome of what you will see (i.e., the likelihood of distress). Because these LLMs assess the harmlessness of content, social media platforms can avoid serving you harmful content.

Running machine learning models to scan content

Social media apps also constantly run machine learning models to scan content for signs of suicide or self-harm by identifying patterns associated with self-harm or suicide ideation. If such signs are detected, users can be flagged as potential beneficiaries of an intervention. Social media platforms are more than ever conscious of compliance requirements. The auditing and transparency tools that social media platforms use can ensure algorithms do not push harmful material and that the embedded safety features are working as intended. These can make social media platforms accountable. Also, as discussed before, social media platforms have automated moderation systems that can make use of machine learning and natural language processing (NLP) to detect content that may violate policies or community standards, such as hate speech, violence, or abusive language.

How to reduce your exposure to harmful content

Leverage the "Not Interested" feature

Some harmful content may slip through content moderation and classification systems. In such cases, if a user has viewed a harmful post, such as an image of self-injury, chances are that the social media algorithms will push them more similar content, because, as mentioned before, social media algorithms are designed to increase engagement. If this happens and you see harmful content on your screen, click the "Not Interested" button to let the social media algorithm know your preference. You can also turn on the social media filters available to you. These can block content you deem sensitive or unsafe from showing up in your social media feed. But these filters tend to be "opt-in" rather than "opt-out". That is, their default setting is not "opt-out", but instead "opt-in", so you need to make an active choice to prevent harmful content like pornography from being displayed in your feed.

Scroll fast through undesirable content and diversify your feed

Watching images of young people with exceptionally fit bodies who lead idealised lifestyles can cause unhealthy social comparisons. The unrealistic standards they set can worsen your body image, which can lead to disordered eating. Social media users often post their best images, not their real ones, after filtering, editing, and AI-altering them. Because the social media algorithm has noticed that you engaged with this content, it will serve you more of it. The best thing to do in this case is to scroll as fast as you can the second the post appears, which will signal to the social media algorithm that you are not interested in this content. Another thing you can do, as mentioned before, is to diversify your feed by seeking information on a completely different topic.

Set boundaries and reduce emotional overload

Passive scrolling of your favourite social media feeds can't fulfil a meaningful human connection. Similarly, online ties don't provide the quality of interaction that face-to-face interaction with friends does. In fact, heavy social media use can replace offline activities like face-to-face socialising, which can worsen your feelings of isolation. Also, some online relationships can be unhealthy or, worse, toxic or manipulative. Being ghosted, blocked, or unfollowed can feel like rejection. Social media apps, such as WhatsApp, analyse not only content, but also interaction. For example, if they detect a user constantly messaging another, demanding their attention, they can flag this interaction pattern. To avoid pressure, set boundaries, and reduce emotional overload, you can mute users, limit their DMs, and restrict who can contact you.

What to do if your social media or online relationships are not healthy

Chris didn't realise he had lost control until social media started controlling his mood, confidence, and time. If your online life feels more draining than uplifting, it's a sign that something needs to change, and there are clear steps you can take to fix it.

1 Manage risks about who you interact with

The internet makes it easy to meet new people, but not everyone online is genuine. Some may pretend to be someone they're not or try to get information from you. Being smart about who you talk to helps you stay safe while still enjoying the fun and connection that social media offers. Staying safe online isn't about cutting off social media completely. It's about using the tools available to protect yourself.

Remember that people lie:

- ☑ Remember that most people online are not who they say they are.
- ☑ Unless you have met someone offline, always assume people may be hiding behind fake profiles, so avoid oversharing.
- ☑ If you're connecting with someone new, a quick video call helps confirm they're real.

Protect your privacy:

- ☑ Use your privacy settings to keep everything private and limit who can see your content and who can contact you.
- ☑ Pause before posting and ask, "Would I be okay if this were shared publicly?"
- ☑ Mute or block a contact when you feel uncomfortable, as this will protect your mental space. Blocking isn't rude, it's healthy.

2 Respect consent in digital spaces

Consent isn't just a real-life concept, as it's equally important online. Respecting boundaries relating to messages, pictures, and personal space is part of being a good digital friend. You also deserve to have your own boundaries respected without guilt or pressure.

You must never share anyone's pictures, videos, or private messages without permission. If someone says "no" to talking, sharing, or meeting, respect it. Silence doesn't mean yes, and you shouldn't keep messaging someone who isn't replying.

You also must remember your right to say no. You don't owe anyone replies, selfies, or constant access to your time.

3 Focus on healthy online and offline friendships and relationships

Online friendships and relationships can feel just as real as offline ones. They can give you support, fun, and even a safe place to be yourself. But just like in-person relationships, the healthy ones make you feel good about yourself, and the unhealthy ones leave you feeling drained or upset.

Ensure you balance online and offline interactions. Digital connections are great, but real-life bonds matter too and are extremely important for your health. Offline interactions are much more effective at making you feel socially connected and less lonely than online interactions.

Look for mutual effort and authenticity with your online relationships. Healthy relationships involve give-and-take and not one person doing all the giving or chasing. Ensure you feel you can be your authentic self. It's tempting to show a perfect version of yourself, but honest connections last longer and are much more meaningful.

> **Check how it feels when you interact with someone**: Do you feel supported, respected, and accepted? Or anxious, pressured, and drained? *That's your red flag test.*

4 Watch out for harmful uses of social media

Social media can be fun and exciting, but it's also designed to play tricks on your brain. The more you compare yourself to others or chase likes, the worse you may feel. Being aware of these traps helps you step back and protect your mental health. Watch out for the following traps that can be detrimental to your mental health and well-being:

- ☑ **Comparison trap:** Remember, you're seeing highlight reels or pictures, not what their life is really like
- ☑ **FOMO:** Just because others post fun moments doesn't mean you're missing something in your life or need to see more of someone else's life
- ☑ **Self-validation:** If your mood depends on how many likes or comments you get, take a step back, as your worth isn't measured by this
- ☑ **Stuck in echo chambers:** Algorithms feed you more of what you engage with, so be aware of how this can distort the reality of what you think and feel

5 Protect your mental health

Your mental health matters as much online as offline. Too much screen time, negative content, or toxic relationships can wear you down. You should ensure you have effective strategies to help you keep control, so social media and online relationships enrich your life rather than drain it. Consider strategies like:

- ☑ **Set limits:** Use app timers or screen time trackers to avoid endless scrolling
- ☑ **Take breaks:** Try staying off social media for 24 hours to recharge and help reset your brain
- ☑ **Manage your feed:** Follow accounts that inspire, educate, or make you feel good and unfollow or block what fuels insecurity or gets you emotional
- ☑ **Check how you feel:** After scrolling, ask "Do I feel better or worse?", if worse, then it's time for a break

Ensure you reach out if social media or online relationships are causing you distress. If online life feels overwhelming, talk to a trusted friend, parent, or school official. You can also call anonymous helplines if you need to talk to someone and are worried about being judged.

Search online for "kids helpline [your country]"; "teen mental health helpline"; "youth crisis line"

Conclusion

Social media affects how you feel about yourself and can have a big impact on your mental health. Online friendships and relationships can be fun, but they also come with risks. These risks relate to people not being honest, pressuring you, or taking advantage of your trust. This chapter helps you navigate all of that. You'll get practical tips for staying safe online, spotting the harmful effects of social media, like comparing yourself to everyone else, and keeping your interactions healthy. You'll also learn how to understand consent in online conversations, protect yourself from exploitation, and build real, positive connections with others. On top of that, this chapter gives tools and strategies to handle stress, reduce the negative impacts of scrolling, and make your time online work for you, not against you.

Key terms

- Social media
- Online relationships
- Self-harm
- Harmful content
- Algorithms
- Social comparison
- Disordered eating
- Loneliness
- Social disconnection
- Online social support
- Dopamine
- Online self-presentation

Bibliography

American Psychological Association. (2025, June 9). *Screen time problems in children*. https://www.apa.org/news/press/releases/2025/06/screen-time-problems-children

Alter, C. (2025, June 18). *Social media case involving Instagram and TikTok*. Time. https://time.com/7295323/social-media-case-instagram-tiktok/

Alter, C. (2025, August 20). *Instagram lawsuit over self-harm content*. Time. https://time.com/7310444/instagram-lawsuit-self-harm/

Anderson, M., & Jiang, J. (2018, November 28). *Teens, social media and technology*. Pew Research Center. https://www.pewresearch.org/internet/2018/11/28/teens-social-media-habits-and-experiences/

Australian Institute of Family Studies. (2021, August 5). *Too much time on screens*. https://aifs.gov.au/resources/short-articles/too-much-time-screens

Berry, S. (2025, April 29). *"I fall asleep in class": New program to tackle teen screen habits*. The Sydney Morning Herald. https://www.smh.com.au/lifestyle/health-and-wellness/i-fall-asleep-in-class-new-program-to-tackle-teen-s-screen-habits-20250428-p5lupq.html

Black Dog Institute. (n.d.). *Links between screen time and depression in adolescents are more complex than first thought*. https://www.blackdoginstitute.org.au/news/links-between-screen-time-and-depression-in-adolescents-more-complex-than-first-thought/

Bowman, A. (2023, September 5). *Social media's effects on the teen brain*. Mayo Clinic. https://mcpress.mayoclinic.org/parenting/social-media-affects-teens-brains/

Bozzola, E., Spina, G., Agostiniani, R., Barni, S., Russo, R., Scarpato, E., Di Mauro, A., Di Stefano, A.V., Caruso, C., Corsello, G., & Staiano, A. (2022). The use of social media in children and adolescents: Scoping review on the potential risks. *International Journal of Environmental Research and Public Health*, *19*(16), 9960. https://doi.org/10.3390/ijerph19169960

Columbia University Mailman School of Public Health. (2021, September 27). *Just how harmful is social media? Our experts weigh in*. https://www.publichealth.columbia.edu/news/just-how-harmful-social-media-our-experts-weigh

De, D., El Jamal, M., Aydemir, E., & Khera, A. (2025). Social media algorithms and teen addiction: Neurophysiological impact and ethical considerations. *Cureus*, *17*(1), e77145. https://doi.org/10.7759/cureus.77145

Department of Infrastructure, Transport, Regional Development, Communications and the Arts. (2023). *Online safety issues survey: Summary report (June 2023)*. Australian Government. https://www.infrastructure.gov.au/sites/default/files/documents/2023-online-safety-issues-survey-summary-report-june2023.pdf

Faverio, M. (2025, July 10). *10 facts about teens and social media*. Pew Research Center. https://www.pewresearch.org/short-reads/2025/07/10/10-facts-about-teens-and-social-media/

Faverio, M., & Sidoti, O. (2025, December 9). *Teens and social media fact sheet*. Pew Research Center. https://www.pewresearch.org/internet/fact-sheet/teens-and-social-media-fact-sheet/

Gerson, J. (2023, September 13). *The complicated ties between teenage girls and social media—and what parents should know*. The 19th News. https://19thnews.org/2023/09/social-media-teenage-girls-mental-health-body-image/

Haidt, J., & Rausch, Z. (2026). Social media is harming adolescents at a scale large enough to cause changes at the population level. In *World Happiness Report 2026* (Chap. 3). https://doi.org/10.18724/WHR-G490-BG86

Hall, R. (2025, August 19). *Social media still pushing suicide-related content to teens despite new UK safety laws*. The Guardian. https://www.theguardian.com/technology/2025/aug/19/social-media-still-pushing-suicide-related-content-to-teens-despite-new-uk-safety-laws

Khalaf, A.M., Alubied, A.A., Khalaf, A.M., & Rifaey, A.A. (2023). The impact of social media on the mental health of adolescents and young adults: A systematic review. *Cureus*, *15*(8), e42990. https://doi.org/10.7759/cureus.42990

Kumar, N. (2025, October 8). *Social media addiction statistics 2025 (trends & facts)*. Demandsage. https://www.demandsage.com/social-media-addiction-statistics/

Lavoipierre, A. (2024, June 2). *Is social media (Facebook and Instagram) linked to teen mental health?* Australian Broadcasting Corporation. https://www.abc.net.au/news/2024-06-02/is-social-media-facebook-instagram-linked-to-teen-mental-health/103838726

Lenharo, M. (2025, May 5). *Young people with internalising disorders and social media sensitivity*. Nature. https://www.nature.com/articles/d41586-025-01359-7

McMahan, I., & Docter Loeb, H. (2025, June 30). *Cellphone addiction, social media and suicidal thoughts among teens*. Washington Post. https://www.washingtonpost.com/wellness/2025/06/30/cellphone-addiction-social-media-suicidal-thoughts/

Maclean, J. (2026). Instagram photo sharing and loneliness differential reactivity: Exploring the moderating effects of online interaction quality and quantity.

International Journal of Human–Computer Interaction, 42(2), 741–751. https://doi.org/10.1080/10447318.2025.2513033

Maclean, J., Al-Saggaf, Y., & Hogg, R. (2022). Instagram photo sharing and its relationships with social connectedness, loneliness, and well-being. *Social Media and Society, 8*(2), 1–13. https://doi.org/10.1177/20563051221107650

Mardon, C. (2024, September 7). *Don't hit publish: Creeps lurking to pinch innocent pics, warns AFP.* News Corp Australia. https://www.news.com.au/technology/online/social/dont-hit-publish-creeps-lurking-to-pinch-innocent-pics-warns-afp-as-sex-exploitation-rises-by-41-per-cent/news-story/cb9121c76fc42ab3628ae5b9234cfd5

Miller, C. (2026, May 6). *Is social media use causing depression?* Child Mind Institute. https://childmind.org/article/is-social-media-use-causing-depression/

Muppalla, S.K., Vuppalapati, S., Reddy Pulliahgaru, A., & Sreenivasulu, H. (2023). Effects of excessive screen time on child development: An updated review and strategies for management. *Cureus, 15*(6), e40608. https://doi.org/10.7759/cureus.40608

OECD. (2026). *Child, adolescent and youth mental health in the 21st century*, OECD Publishing, Paris, https://doi.org/10.1787/1092c3cb-en

Santos, R.M.S., Mendes, C.G., Sen Bressani, G. *et al.* (2023). The associations between screen time and mental health in adolescents: A systematic review. *BMC Psychology, 11*, 127. https://doi.org/10.1186/s40359-023-01166-7

Scott, S. (2022, October 4). *Mental health and teens: Screens research.* Australian Broadcasting Corporation. https://www.abc.net.au/news/2022-10-04/mental-health-teens-screens-research/101495990

Skopeliti, C., Milmo, D., & Skopeliti, C. (2021, September 18). *'I felt my body wasn't good enough': Teenage troubles with Instagram.* The Guardian https://www.theguardian.com/society/2021/sep/18/i-felt-my-body-wasnt-good-enough-teenage-troubles-with-instagram

University of Edinburgh. (2024, January 15). *Teens who increase screen time raise mental health risks.* https://www.ed.ac.uk/news/2024/teens-who-up-screen-time-raise-mental-health-risks

University of Queensland. (2021, August 10). *Excess screen time impacting teen mental health.* https://news.uq.edu.au/2021-08-10-excess-screen-time-impacting-teen-mental-health

Verduyn, P., Gugushvili, N., Massar, K., Täht, K., & Kross, E. (2020). Social comparison on social networking sites. *Current Opinion in Psychology, 36*, 62–66. https://doi.org/10.1016/j.copsyc.2020.04.002

Vogels, E.A., & Gelles-Watnick, R. (2023, April 24). *Teens and social media: Key findings from surveys.* Pew Research Center. https://www.pewresearch.org/short-reads/2023/04/24/teens-and-social-media-key-findings-from-pew-research-center-surveys

Wen, H., Kong, X., & Feng, Y. (2022). The relationship between cyber upward social comparison and cyberbullying behaviors: A moderated mediating model. *Frontiers in Psychology, 13*, 1017775. https://doi.org/10.3389/fpsyg.2022.1017775

Wilksch, S.M., O'Shea, A., Ho, P., Byrne, S., & Wade, T.D. (2020). The relationship between social media use and disordered eating in young adolescents. *International Journal of Eating Disorders, 53*(1), 96–106. https://doi.org/10.1002/eat.23198

World Health Organization. (2024, September 25). *Teens, screens and mental health.* https://www.who.int/europe/news/item/25-09-2024-teens--screens-and-mental-health

Conclusion

The internet can be incredible for building knowledge and connecting with others, but it is not always safe or harmless. Not managing the risks is how you put yourself at risk. What makes the difference is awareness, confidence, and action.

This book has shown you how online harm happens from your digital footprint, smartphone settings, online cyber threats, cyberbullying, trolling and cyberstalking, to sextortion, catfishing, grooming, radicalisation, misinformation, and hate speech. These aren't rare events. They are common tactics used in predictable ways that can be devastating if you don't protect yourself. The ways people manipulate, exploit, deceive, and harm online can be subtle and by the time you notice it can be too late. This book has outlined how you can learn to recognise warning signs, defend yourself, and take back control of your online presence.

The final and most powerful message is that you are fully in control. You can equip yourself with the tools, the awareness, and the ability to shape your digital world into a safer, kinder, and more authentic space, for yourself and for others.

Be aware that everything you are doing is being tracked

Who tracks your online movements, and what information is collected about you?

- Online cookies track what websites you visit
- Applications track everything about you
- Search engines track everything you search for
- Social media tracks every interaction
- Internet service providers track all your online activities

How can you minimise your digital footprint across all the digital channels you use?

- Manage your cookies
- Turn on browser blocker extensions

DOI: 10.4324/9781003681731-14

- Use a Virtual Private Network (VPN)
- Adjust social media privacy settings
- Ensure good password practices
- Stop using your real name publicly online or through your smartphone settings

Your smartphone is powerful, but it can put you at risk

How does your smartphone leak your identifying information?

- Snap Map allows others to track your location
- Apps can share your location data
- Wi-Fi can leak your personal information
- Bluetooth sensors can detect your location
- The microphone and camera can be accessed if not properly secured

How can you secure your smartphone?

- Manage location settings
- Secure Wi-Fi and Bluetooth settings
- Lock down your microphone and camera settings
- Check your other key smartphone privacy settings

Ensure you adopt a zero-trust approach and verify EVERYTHING

How do you protect yourself from how cyber-attacks are executed?

- Spoofing makes it easy to pretend to be someone legitimate
- Be aware of how Typosquatting, Man-in-the-Middle (MITM), and identity theft make it hard to tell if it's not legitimate
- Use trusted apps from verified providers
- Never click on links in SMS or emails
- Always enable multi-factor authentication (MFA)
- Never share your personal details online

How to critically assess information to determine credibility

- Use cross-referencing to validate information
- Always start with the assumption that the information cannot be trusted
- Train yourself to spot fake videos or accounts
- Treat unexpected messages, links, or attachments as suspicious by default
- Check email addresses, usernames, and subtle impersonation signs
- Look for urgency, threats, or pressure tactics commonly used in phishing and scams

- Avoid clicking any links and inspect URLs to confirm legitimacy
- Be cautious of messages asking for personal, financial, or account information

How attackers/predators/perpetrators target you online

Cyberbullying and trolling: Perpetrators seek attention, reaction, or control. They may provoke, harass, or publicly shame to trigger emotional responses or escalate conflict.

Cyberstalking and doxing: They gather personal information over time, sometimes from small details you share, to monitor, intimidate, or expose your location.

Sextortion, catfishing, and grooming: Most cases involve fake or deceptive profiles. They build trust through compliments, attention, or emotional support, then shift to manipulation, isolation, or pressure.

How attackers use technology to target you

- Nearly all cases involve fake profiles
- They usually start with compliments, offers, or by trying to gain your trust
- They will often try to take you to apps or platforms where interactions can't be traced
- They will try to hack your email and password to get access to private photos or videos
- They will use the information they obtained to blackmail you

How to use technical solutions to protect yourself from falling victim to online harm

- Ensure effective management of privacy settings, lock everything down
- Share information carefully to make it difficult for someone to gather information about you
- Use unique and long passwords and avoid using dictionary passwords
- Enable multi-factor authentication (MFA)
- Browse the web securely; use freely available secure browsers
- Remove location or metadata from your posts
- Use safety features to block, report, and document harmful behaviour

How to recognise and protect yourself from problematic situations online

- Recognise and be aware of fake profiles
- Be cautious of unknown accounts
- Manage online friendships safely
- Watch out for things that escalate quickly or feel too intense
- Identify and address uncomfortable online interactions
- Understand and respect consent
- Use reverse image search to catch a catfish or a fake profile

It is too easy to fall victim to harmful online content

How does technology make hate speech and radicalisation worse for young people?

- Algorithms promote radicalisation by repeating similar content and reinforcing extreme view
- Radicals use technology to create the us against them narrative
- Personalised feeds create echo chambers and limit different perspectives
- Constant exposure can make harmful beliefs seem normal or widely accepted
- Online groups use technology to spread us vs them narratives
- Anonymity lowers accountability, increasing hostile and extreme behaviour

How to reduce your exposure to harmful content

- Leverage the "Not Interested" feature
- Scroll fast through undesirable content and diversify your feed
- Set boundaries and reduce emotional overload
- Critically assess information you see online
- Implement content moderation and content classification to reduce exposure
- Run machine learning models to scan content
- Use sophisticated search queries to validate information
- Be aware of how censorship, deplatforming, and content moderation increase misinformation

Gaming, Social Media, and AI: Powerful tools with real risks

How to protect yourself in online gaming and social platforms

- Recognise that harmful behaviour in online spaces is often driven by reward through attention, control, or reaction
- Use strong, unique passwords to secure your accounts
- Maximise privacy settings to limit who can contact or view you
- Choose platforms that actively detect bullying
- Take advantage of built-in safety features
- Use device and platform controls to manage screen time and reduce overuse

How to manage social comparison on social media

- Remind yourself that what you see online is selective, edited, and often unrealistic
- Avoid measuring your worth against someone else's highlight reel
- Be mindful of how certain content makes you feel
- Unfollow or mute accounts that negatively impact your well-being

How to recognise the influence of AI Chatbots

- Set clear boundaries for how and when you use AI tools
- Use smartphone digital well-being features to reduce distractions and overreliance
- Follow age-based guidelines to ensure safe and appropriate use
- Build awareness of how AI systems are designed to build emotional connection so you can engage with them critically

Follow the SAFE method if something feels wrong online

S – Stop all contact

Pause straight away. Don't reply, don't click links, and don't send anything back.

A – Assess the risk

Think it through by asking, does this feel safe or right? Trust your instincts. If something feels off, it probably is.

F – Focus on protecting yourself

Take control of the situation:

- Save evidence (screenshots, messages, usernames)
- Block the person or account
- Report the behaviour on the platform
- Avoid further contact or engagement

E – Engage support

Reach out to someone you trust through a parent, caregiver, teacher, or another safe adult. Search online for your countries support services as there is a lot of good online and phone resources specifically for teens. You don't have to handle it alone. Adults want to help and support you.

Be part of protecting other teens online

Online safety is not only about protecting yourself. It is also about looking out for the people around you. The way you act online can genuinely change someone else's experience, sometimes more than you realise.

Being someone who makes a positive difference looks like:

- Be a voice that lifts others up
- Don't spread harm or negativity

- Speak up when something doesn't feel right
- Share what you know to help others stay safe
- Lead by example
- Be an upstander, not a bystander

You must always:

- Report hate or harassment even if it's not aimed at you
- Check in on someone who seems upset or targeted
- Refuse to like, share, or pass on harmful content
- Talk with your friends about what they're experiencing online

Every time you choose kindness, respect, and responsibility, you make the internet safer for yourself and for everyone around you.

Final thoughts

Cyber threats thrive in silence. By reporting and taking action, you protect yourself, limit damage, and stop attackers from harming others. Managing your digital footprint and being proactive about security not only shields you from risks now but also builds a safe, positive online presence for your future.

You cannot control every risk online. No one can. But you can control how you respond. You can manage your privacy settings. You can question suspicious content. You can verify before you click. You can refuse to share personal information. You can walk away from harmful spaces. Those small, consistent actions build real protection.

The goal is not to fear the internet. It is to understand it. When you understand how risks work, you reduce their power. When you stay alert, informed, and proactive, you stay in control.

If you are a parent, caregiver, teacher, or anyone that cares about teens

Supporting teens in the digital world begins with creating a genuinely safe space grounded in trust, open communication, and empathy. Whether you're a parent, carer, teacher, or simply someone who cares about young people, your role is more influential than you might realise.

Consider the following approaches:

1. Keep communication open and ongoing
2. Listen first before reacting or problem-solving
3. Focus on teaching skills, not just enforcing rules
4. Model healthy and respectful online behaviour
5. Encourage critical thinking and self-protection
6. Stay informed about emerging digital trends and risks
7. Build a network of trusted adults around them

8 Reinforce that they are never alone
9 Promote kindness, accountability, and responsibility
10 Respond early and supportively to warning signs

Remember that the most powerful protection you can offer a teen is your consistent presence. Showing up calmly, reliably, and without judgement creates the foundation they need to feel safe.

Teens need to know that no matter what happens online, they won't have to face it alone. Whether they've made a mistake, been hurt, or simply don't know what to do next, your steady support can give them the confidence to speak up and the resilience to move forward.

In a digital world that can be both challenging and full of opportunity, your presence matters more than any rule, app, or monitoring tool. It's what ultimately helps young people not just stay safe online, but truly develop resilience to harm.

Index

For Product Safety Concerns and Information please contact our EU representative GPSR@taylorandfrancis.com Taylor & Francis Verlag GmbH, Kaufingerstraße 24, 80331 München, Germany